Tra

Den

Through the TTAP Method

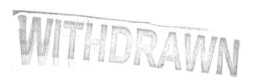

Additional TTAP Method® Resources

By Linda Levine Madori, Ph.D., CTRS, ATR-BC

PUBLICATION

Therapeutic Thematic Arts Programming for Older Adults

This introduction to the TTAP Method® describes powerful programming and benefits for well elders and those facing illness or disability.

Available at http://www.healthpropress.com/ttap

EDUCATIONAL DVDs

See the TTAP Method® in action in live sessions with long-term care residents.

Meditation, Storytelling, and Poetry Program

Mask-Making Program

Creating a Bird Nest Sculpture

Available at http://www.healthpropress.com/ttap

PROFESSIONAL TRAINING

TTAP Method® Certification Courses available for staff, professionals, and researchers

plus

TTAP Method® Overview for Alzheimer's Care

and

TTAP Method® for Caregivers

Visit http://www.healthpropress.com/training for more information

Transcending Dementia

Through the TTAP Method

A New Psychology of Art, Brain, and Cognition

by

Linda Levine Madori,
Ph.D., CTRS, ATR-BC

Foreword by
Christopher S. Nadeau,
M.S., QDCS, TTAP-C

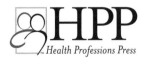

HPP
Health Professions Press

Baltimore • London • Sydney

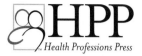

Health Professions Press, Inc.
Post Office Box 10624
Baltimore, Maryland 21285-0624
www.healthpropress.com

TTAP Method® is a trademark of Linda Levine Madori.

Art on the cover copyright © 2012 by Linda Levine Madori.

Typeset by Barton Matheson Willse & Worthington, Baltimore, Maryland.
Cover design by Mindy Dunn.
Manufactured in the United States of America by Versa Press, East Peoria, Illinois.

The information provided in this book is in no way meant to substitute for a medical practitioner's advice or expert opinion. Readers should consult a medical professional if they are interested in more information. This book is sold without warranties of any kind, express or implied, and the publisher and author disclaim any liability, loss, or damage caused by the contents of this book.

Library of Congress Cataloging-in-Publication data

Levine Madori, Linda.
   Transcending dementia through the TTAP method / by Linda Levine Madori :
foreword by Christopher S. Nadeau.
      p. cm.
   Includes bibliographical references and index.
   ISBN 978-1-932529-72-2 (pbk.)
   I. Title.
   [DNLM: 1. Alzheimer Disease—therapy.   2. Art Therapy—methods.
3. Dementia—therapy.   WT 155]

   616.89'1656—dc23

                                                                      2012026970

British Cataloguing in Publication data are available from the British Library.

Contents

About the Author   vii

Foreword, by Christopher Nadeau   ix

Preface   xiii

Acknowledgments   xvii

Introduction   1

Chapter 1   Overview of Alzheimer's Disease   7

Chapter 2   Overview of the Therapeutic Thematic Arts
            Programming Method   25

Chapter 3   TTAP Method Programming for People with
            Alzheimer's Disease   43

Chapter 4   Brain Functioning, Cognition, and the
            TTAP Method   87

Chapter 5   Using the TTAP Method to Stimulate Cognitive
            Functioning   103

Chapter 6   Aging and Human Developmental Theories:
            Understanding and Meeting the Needs of
            Older Adults, Including Those with Dementia   121

Chapter 7   Documentation and Replication of Research on
            the TTAP Method   157

Appendix A   Program Protocols for the TTAP Method   173
Appendix B   TTAP Method Activity Assessment Form   189
Appendix C   Sources for Art Supplies and Music   197
Appendix D   Graphic Organizing Tools   207
Appendix E   Themes in the TTAP Method   215

References   217
Index   233

About the Author

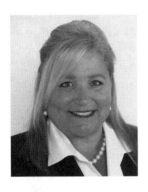

Linda Levine Madori, Ph.D., CTRS, ATR-BC, is a professor at St. Thomas Aquinas College in Sparkill, New York, where she has taught therapeutic recreation and creative arts therapies since 1996. She also has a private practice and lives in Westchester, New York. Since 1984, Dr. Levine Madori has worked in the field of health care as a therapist, teacher, advisor, and researcher. She received her Ph.D. in health education studies from New York University. Her dissertation, *Cognitive and Psychosocial Functioning in Residents with Alzheimer's Disease: Therapeutic Recreation Participation Correlated to Improved Cognition and Quality of Life in Those Residents Living in a Skilled Nursing Facility* (2009), is the basis for her first book, *Therapeutic Thematic Arts Programming for Older Adults* (Health Professions Press, 2007).

Since the publication of her first book, Dr. Levine Madori has received two Fulbright Scholarships in Global Health (2007 & 2009) to teach her innovative method internationally in Australia, New Zealand, and Finland. She has received awards at the national and state level for the TTAP Method® for "Best Practice Approach" to dementia care. Dr. Levine Madori has also established an international affiliation through St. Thomas Aquinas College with HAMK University of Applied Sciences in Finland. Each year students from the college can register to take a course in Therapeutic Thematic Arts Programming (TTAP Method) in Finland with students from all over Europe.

Dr. Levine Madori holds credentials in both therapeutic recreation (M.S.) and art therapy (ATR-BC) and is licensed in the state of New York in creative arts therapy (ATR-BC#000971-1). She has had the unique experience of being professionally active on the state level as well as internationally in moving therapeutic recreation and art therapy forward into the 21st century. She has chaired the Leisure and

Aging Track of the American Society on Aging; served on the Leisure and Aging Section of the National Recreation and Park Association; and served as Master Supervisor for the American Art Therapy Association, developing professional educational intensives for the Society on Arts in Healthcare, the Veteran's Association of Hospitals Nationwide, the American Art Therapy Association, and the American Therapeutic Recreation Association. Dr. Levine Madori has been a keynote presenter for the International Alzheimer's Association, the International Creative Expression Communication and Dementia (CECD) Conference, the Edna Gates Foundation, and other prestigious state, national, and international organizations.

Therapeutic Thematic Arts Programming for Older Adults was translated into Finnish in 2009 through HAMK University Press. To date, 11 studies conducted in the United States, Finland, and Australia have demonstrated the efficacy of this structured multimodal approach, which has been proven effective with many varied populations, including children, adolescents, and adults with autism, developmental disabilities, and psychiatric disorders.

In 2009, Dr. Levine Madori launched a 2-day (14-hour, CEU-approved) TTAP Method Certification Training Program. She conducts both national and international trainings through the National Fulbright Office, the New York State Office on Aging, Beth Abraham Hospital and Family Services, and Linden Oaks at Edward Hospital as well as universities throughout the state of New York. TTAP Method Certification Training is also available through the Seminars on Site program offered by Health Professions Press, Inc. (https://www.health propress.com/training).

For more information on how you can take a course in the TTAP Method, to receive certification in the TTAP Method, or to arrange for a certification training at your facility or organization, contact seminars@healthpropress.com. Dr. Levine Madori can be contacted at Linda@Levinemadoriphd.com.

Foreword

Once considered a rare disorder, this thief of memory we call Alzheimer's disease is taking over our communities and compromising the ability of families to live at home with dignity. More than 15 million people care for someone with memory loss; their unpaid care services have a yearly value of over $202 billion to the nation; and the annual cost to U.S. businesses is estimated at over $61 billion. In 2012, every 69 seconds someone in America develops Alzheimer's disease and one in every two residents over the age of 80 in a nursing home has some form of dementia. The disease is now the sixth-leading cause of death for those over the age of 65.

The challenges of caring for adults with Alzheimer's disease brings into sharp focus the many issues we are facing as a nation around the delivery of quality health care and other services for an aging population. Serving on several different boards and as a long-time organizer and advocate for social insurance, entitlement, and long-term care reform—I am deeply involved in the dialogue about what is at stake for older Americans:

It's the spring of 1999, and I'm sitting in a press conference strategy meeting on Capitol Hill for a Pew Charitable Trust national education campaign, "Americans Discuss Social Security." The youthful, newly elected mayor of Valente, New York, leans over and says to me, "We must ensure a good quality of life for our seniors." I nod. The next morning the Mayor and I are in the halls of Congress, standing before a large podium. Senator Charles Grassley, Chairman of the Special Committee on Aging, stands between us wrapping up his speech by saying, "Our seniors deserve a dignified retirement and quality of life." I agree and then deliver my own speech. A year later I'm moderating a panel discussion on health and life issues for a large Generation X national advocacy convention in Philadelphia. The last person on the panel is Dr. Baruch Blumberg, the 1976 winner of the Nobel Prize for Medicine and current Director of NASA's Astrobiology Institute. He ends his presentation with a similar statement and espouses the bioethical value and benefits of upholding a good quality of life for seniors in need of medical services.

It is a recurrent theme, this search for quality in long-term care in general and in Alzheimer's care most emphatically. A critical piece of this conversation about quality care is the inherent correlation between cost and access to care, which at the start of the 21st century has become impossible to ignore. Between 1960 and 2008, health care spending as a percentage of gross national product went from 5% to more than 16%. From 1998 to 2008, average health insurance premiums and worker contributions for family coverage more than doubled. Given the tsunami of baby boomers who will reach retirement years within the next few decades, the challenge of maintaining, much less improving, the overall quality of care looms large. We must ask ourselves if all of this spending is translating into a health care system we want for ourselves, our loved ones, and the communities we live in.

Finding more affordable care practices that do not compromise, and that in fact enhance, quality of life is our new imperative. Dr. Linda Levine Madori's Therapeutic Thematic Arts Programming Method (TTAP Method®) is one such alternative. It is a refreshing contribution to the science of health and well-being for those who are living with memory loss, offering a profound revelation as to the potential impact we can have in the lives of people living with the disease. The operative word here is *living,* and if anything comes of what we know today about treating the symptoms of Alzheimer's disease and related dementias, it is that social constructs are not only necessary but mandatory in supporting an individual's desire to have a life worth living. Grounded in current brain research, the TTAP Method is a powerfully effective way of using the creative arts, meditation, and social interaction to stimulate mental functioning and increase each person's sense of self-efficacy and self-worth despite the losses from a debilitating disease. There is life after diagnosis and the TTAP Method supports the capacity a person retains in all domains of health and well-being: psychological, social, spiritual, cognitive, and physical. Of equal value, the method provides structure and direction to the therapist or caregiver.

Imagine if you will that as early as 5,000 B.C.E. various healing traditions recognized the body, mind, and spirit connection, and that health was viewed within the purview of balancing these three in harmony within the free flow of invisible vital energy referred to as *qi* in China or *prana* in India. In her pioneering TTAP Method, Dr. Levine Madori bridges the divide between Old World thinking, modern neuroscience, and cutting-edge arts-based programming in a way that places cognitive and physical engagement firmly within the constructs of human wellness.

In the absence of a cure, the TTAP Method offers the potential to save our Alzheimer's health care system billions of dollars. Dr. Levine Madori is part of a new wave of thinkers who are helping professionals in the long-term care field begin to shift and realize that access to this new paradigm of medical care transcends the boundaries between health and social care. Here is a vital force for ensuring personal responsibility and personal transformation by peeling away the surface of an outdated, over-medicalized, costly, and underperforming health care system. In just one setting, at a Chicago nursing home, the TTAP Method was shown to reduce the need for nursing care by more than 50% while at the same time improving care quality and satisfaction.

I am Executive Director of the New York Memory Center in Brooklyn, New York, a national model program for social adult day centers in the United States that is often visited by scholars, administrators, and health care practitioners from places as far off as Japan and Australia. We embrace the latest evidenced-based and evidenced-informed nonpharmacological approaches to wellness, including arts-based programming; cognitive stimulation; exercise and movement training; meditation; learning methods; sensory therapy; cognitive training; tailored diets; communication techniques for managing behavioral symptoms; early stage education and peer support designed to maximize independence and reduce excess disability; and caregiver education, coaching, counseling, and advanced care planning. Our team has seen first-hand how the TTAP Method has enhanced our own care model. We see deeper and more meaningful levels of bonding between peers and overall enhanced cohesion among-and-between members of the program with various stages of memory loss. We see a faster turnaround from social isolation and depression to active involvement and joyful participation in activities. Some members who did not previously have an interest in the arts or meditation, for example, now willingly enjoy a full day of such programming around a theme, regardless of the activity. Ultimately, our greatest measure of success, which I believe the TTAP Method is supporting, is our continued ability to delay premature institutionalization and to keep families safely together as long as therapeutically possible.

Our society enters the beginning of the 21st century asking new questions about the role of our health care system, recognizing that we must not simply aim to prevent and cure disease but to maintain optimal health. In the face of the economic, medical, and quality-of-life issues that are arising from ever-increasing life spans, we are all the better for Dr. Levine Madori's contributions to the field. Our challenge for the future will be to embrace this method and ensure widespread dissemination within our long-term care system: nursing homes, adult day centers, assisted living, and other settings. If it contributes to maintaining and improving quality of life for older adults, doesn't this reflect the type of health care system we want for ourselves and for society as a whole?

Christopher S. Nadeau, MS, QDCS, TTAP-C
Executive Director
New York Memory Center

Preface

I developed the Therapeutic Thematic Arts Programming Method (or TTAP Method®, pronounced "tap method") from 1986 through 1995, while working at the largest continuum of care facilities for older adults in Riverdale, New York. As both a licensed art therapist and a certified recreation therapist, I had worked full-time serving various populations (roughly 1,500 people), including well older adults, people with Alzheimer's disease (mild, moderate, and severe), and residents in assisted living or skilled nursing care.

While developing the TTAP Method, I have had the unique opportunity to witness a number of benefits for the people I have worked with, including increased social participation, longer periods of time engaging in the activities, higher levels of awareness, and increased positive feelings. Most significant and clearly noticeable was that those who were engaging in creative arts programming were living longer than those who declined to participate. Also, those who lived independently or in an assisted living unit who engaged in the programming formed close ties and relationships with those around them, because the TTAP Method naturally enables group members to share and learn about one another's lives. People living in the Alzheimer's disease units became significantly more fluid in their speech and ability to communicate while participating in the programming than they were at any other time of day. Nursing staff, social workers, and physicians told me that they had no idea the residents in their care could carry on a conversation and interact with those around them, let alone participate in creative arts activities and for long periods of time. In the 1980s and 1990s, recreation therapists and activity professionals were taught that programming for the dementia population should last no longer than 30 minutes. My programs were running longer than 2 hours. At times, the nursing staff had to ask me to end the activities because it was time to serve lunch.

Besides facilitating creative arts programming at the Riverdale facility, I developed meditation and guided imagery sessions for well older adults and meditation programming for people residing in the assisted living and skilled nursing care units. At that time it was unusual to hold a meditation session in a nursing facility, but I was fortunate in that I always involved the nurses in what I was doing. All of the participants who started to do meditations responded positively, with such comments as "I feel better than I have felt all week after this session," "I look forward to these sessions and wouldn't miss them," and "I have my family visit on days that the meditation sessions aren't given, so I don't miss any; this is as important as my medicine." I then began to get other reactions that I had not expected. One woman who had Parkinson's disease joined the group on the advice of her room-mate, and after the session she shared that during the meditation she had not had tremors. Another person who experienced numbness in her arms said that her discomfort subsided while she meditated.

With all this positive feedback, I decided to ask the facility's administration whether I could try to adapt a meditation and guided imagery session for those in the Alzheimer's unit. I clearly remember his response: "People with Alzheimer's can't meditate!" To which I replied, "How do we know they can't? No one has ever tried." And with that, he agreed to allow me to conduct one session to see how it went. The residents were in the mild to moderate stages of the disease, yet they responded positively to the music, and some even closed their eyes for a few minutes and relaxed in their chairs. After the session, I asked the participants what they had seen, if anything, in their mind's eye. The responses overwhelmed me. One woman said that she had seen the mountain house that her family went to in Maine each year and that she had felt as though she was actually there again. This woman had never said more than "yes" or "no" to me. To get such a response was shocking. Another woman stated that she had heard the birds in the music and had seen herself at the beach on the Jersey shore, a favorite place where she had spent her summers.

These experiences made me realize that a relaxation response to music and meditation can be facilitated for all populations, even with those living with Alzheimer's and other dementias. It also allowed me to link the concept of what participants saw in their mind's eye to what they could draw, paint, or sculpt. This was how I initially began to apply a thematic approach to arts programming, and over the years it became clear to me that this approach worked well. It was not until a decade later, however, that I came to truly understand how the TTAP Method works in stimulating various regions of the brain in people with Alzheimer's.

In 1999, I began work on my Ph.D. at New York University. I chose to focus my research on the cognitive and psychological effects that art and recreation therapy were having on those I had been working with. This started my dissertation work, which is titled *Cognitive and Psychosocial Functioning in Residents with Alzheimer's Disease: Therapeutic Recreation Participation Correlated to Improved Cognition and Quality of Life in Those Residents Living in a Skilled Nursing Facility* (Levine Madori, 2009).

I first set out to work with people diagnosed with mild Alzheimer's. However, I had not realized how difficult this task would prove to be. In the United States, as in many other countries, those with mild Alzheimer's are more often cared for at home by family members and with home health care rather than in a skilled nursing facility (SNF). After visiting five SNFs in New York, I eventually found 120 people who had mild Alzheimer's. I measured the amount of time each person spent in art and recreation programming and how often he or she participated in programming against his or her overall psychosocial well-being. My research findings showed significant and positive correlations between the time and frequency spent in arts programming and increased cognition and psychosocial well-being in the 120 participants over the course of their first year in the SNF.

My dissertation was the basis for my first book, *Therapeutic Thematic Arts Programming for Older Adults,* which was published in 2007. Since then, the TTAP Method has been recognized by the Council for International Exchange of Scholars (CIES) as a powerful intervention to change how we care for, interact with, and significantly increase the quality of life for the millions of people diagnosed with Alzheimer's disease. In 2007, CIES gave me the first of two Fulbright Senior Specialist Awards to teach a 6-week course in New Zealand and Australia on this innovative approach to engaging those with Alzheimer's. During this Fulbright term, I was invited to give the keynote address for the International Alzheimer's Conference in Wellington, New Zealand. I also gave lectures in Australia to health care professionals and caregivers as well as to those recently diagnosed with Alzheimer's.

In 2009, I was given a second Fulbright Award to teach the TTAP Method to graduate and undergraduate students in major universities throughout Finland. In addition, the Finnish government requested through the Finnish Fulbright Office that I develop a certificate course on the TTAP Method, which was taught through Seinajoki University, the University of Tampere, the University of Helsinki, and HAMK University Continuing Education Program. Also while in Finland, I was invited to host a half-day teaching seminar through the Finnish Alzheimer's Association in Helsinki.

Since the publication of *Therapeutic Thematic Arts Programming for Older Adults,* 11 studies conducted in the United States, Finland, and Australia have examined the effectiveness of the TTAP Method with different cohorts, from well older adults to people living in assisted living or skilled nursing care to people with Alzheimer's (Alders & Levine Madori, 2010; Hanski & Kahola, 2009; Hemming, 2009; Ketola, 2010; Levine Madori, 2005, 2009a, 2009b; Peltokangus & Rantala, 2009; Vanaska, 2009). Each study showed improved cognitive functioning, both self-perceived by the participants and actual cognitive abilities as observed by staff and researchers, as a result of time spent in structured thematic arts programming (Levine Madori, 2009a,b,c). Interviews with study participants also showed greater feelings of well-being.

As I continue to conduct training on applying the TTAP Method in the United States and internationally, my main objective is to show how the method provides the early intervention needed to assist older adults diagnosed with Alzheimer's and other dementias in retaining cognitive and psychosocial abilities (Blacker et al., 2007; Kinsella et al., 2008). It is my hope that eventually the TTAP Method, at its best, will be used by art and recreation therapists as well as by activity professionals in long-term care, skilled nursing, assisted living, adult day services, and memory care centers in caring for people diagnosed with Alzheimer's or other forms of dementia.

Acknowledgments

I am truly indebted to the following people for their help, support, and belief in my work.

To my husband, Lee, thank you for always being there through thick and thin. You have witnessed the culmination of this massive amount of work over the past 2 years; this manuscript has been on many of our summer and winter vacations. You have always answered whatever questions I have had, helped in solving my problems, and continually respected the work I was destined to do.

To Mary Magnus, Director of Publications at Health Professions Press, for believing in my vision of how arts, the brain, and cognition work together and for sharing my professional adventures over many phone calls and emails throughout the past 7 years and across continents.

To Cecilia González, my developmental editor, who edited, re-edited, and edited again the large body of work that has comprised this new publication. It has been a long time in coming and I could not have gotten here without you and your continual support in reworking my research and thoughts into this comprehensive book. Thank you for being there in my darkest hours and for encouraging me when I thought I could not edit another page!

To my dear friends: Bobbi, Linda, and Leonor, who may have been born from other Mothers, but who are surely my sisters in this lifetime. Thank you all for calling me when I have been overwhelmed, continually comforting me through my life's ebbs and flows, and always sharing good meals with red wine and laughter.

To my students at St. Thomas Aquinas College, from HAMK University, and from the Finnish International Summer School, as well as to those students who have followed me across oceans to Finland—you come into my classrooms ready and willing to share your deepest thoughts and to challenge yourselves through personal discovery. I learn from all of you, and I am deeply blessed to be your teacher, mentor, and professional peer.

To all the health care professionals who have taken my TTAP Method Certification course. We share the same vision—we can change the health care system and we can lessen health care costs by how we communicate with each other and the people we care for through the creative arts. Our government, health care system, and practitioners need to continue to support and fund nonpharmacological approaches that enhance evidence-based research into how the creative arts can improve the cognitive functioning and overall well-being of those we care for as well as reduce health care costs.

Lastly, I want to recognize Dr. Margaret Fitzpatrick, President of St. Thomas Aquinas College. You are my role model and a true visionary in the field of higher education. I have had the pleasure of witnessing over the past 15 years how you have changed the face of our college, erected buildings where there was only dust, created programs to better our community, increased our student body, and enhanced our educational structure. Thank you for always supporting my work at St. Thomas Aquinas and believing in my visions for how we can enhance the aging process.

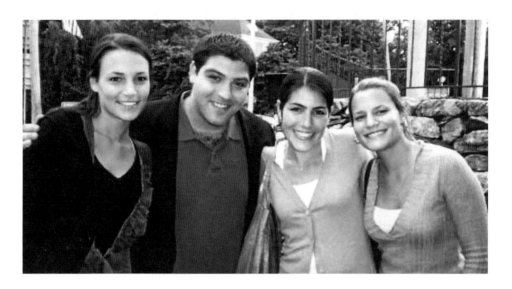

This book is dedicated to my four children,
Lea, Casey, Melanie, and Lorin.

I often tell each of you those three simple words: I love you. What I want each of you to be aware of is just how significantly you all impact my life work, my ability to teach, my desire to travel, my joys, and my passions. I wouldn't be able to do what I do if it weren't for all four of you. I have watched with great pride as each one of you has grown into a successful individual, creating meaningful lives and families of your own.

The most significant role of my life began as mother when each one of you entered my world, and now my journey continues as each of you expands our family with lovers, husbands, and grandchildren. Remember, my children, memories are where immortality exists—it exists when I look into each of your smiling eyes, when you share a brilliant moment of your day, and when I hear your children's laughter.

Lastly, just as my Grandma Betty is alive in my heart and through the stories and memories shared with each of you, remember that now is your time, time to create your own family memories and keep your stories alive. Revisit your favorite memories, share them with those you love, and, most important, laugh as often as you can.

This book is dedicated to each of you
with my deepest love,
Mom

Introduction

The foundations of this book come from more than 30 years of the author's hands-on experience working with older adults as a Certified Recreation Therapist and a Board-Certified Art Therapist. The Therapeutic Thematic Arts Programming Method (TTAP Method™) combines the principles of therapeutic recreation and creative arts therapies into an innovative and person-centered approach to engaging people with Alzheimer's disease and other forms of dementia. Now more than ever before, the creative arts in health care is viewed as a viable intervention for those who are slowly losing functional and cognitive abilities due to a progressive dementia, such as Alzheimer's disease. Anyone who has worked with this population, or who knows someone diagnosed with the disease, knows that the individual can still communicate and engage socially with others, participate in activities, and share personal memories and feelings. Care providers also recognize that certain functional and cognitive strengths and abilities survive throughout the disease process, albeit to a lessening extent.

The TTAP Method draws on the arts by using different forms of creative expression (ranging from music and dance/movement to photography, sculpture, and painting) to build on theme-based activities that can be used to capitalize on remaining strengths and abilities. The programming also provides significant emotional and psychological benefits for participants by creating meaningful outlets for self-expression that can increase feelings of self-worth and self-efficacy. Additional benefits of using the TTAP Method with people with Alzheimer's include multiple opportunities for participants to engage socially, enhanced mood, declines in disruptive behaviors and symptoms of depression, improved memory and recall abilities, and increased use of language.

ABOUT THE BOOK

Chapter 1 provides an overview of Alzheimer's disease, including a discussion of its warning signs and the characteristics of the three main stages of the disease progression (mild, moderate, severe). The chapter also highlights an alternative type of staging based on the individual's remaining strengths and abilities, which the TTAP Method incorporates. Although this book primarily focuses on the role of the therapist in working with people with Alzheimer's, family members can also use the TTAP method to help a loved one diagnosed with Alzheimer's stay connected through words, shared thoughts, and stimulating interactions.

Chapter 2 offers a general overview of the steps of the TTAP Method (which are discussed in more depth in Chapter 3), and begins with a discussion of the value of themes in creative arts therapy. Thematic programming naturally facilitates group activity by continually recognizing and drawing on participants' past and present interests and life experiences. The TTAP Method provides the therapist a structure to explore a theme with a group through different creative arts activities. Chapter highlights also include how the approach incorporates and supports the common strengths and abilities those with Alzheimer's continue to possess throughout the disease process, as well as the concepts promoted by the TTAP Method (personal choice, intrinsic motivation, self-efficacy, and optimal experience [or *flow*]). The TTAP Method as a multimodal care approach and the effectiveness of such approaches for people with Alzheimer's are also covered.

Chapter 3 begins with a discussion of the common communication problems associated with Alzheimer's, and how the TTAP Method addresses them. The therapist begins each creative arts activity with step 1—conversation—as a way to introduce a theme to the group. As participants reflect on a theme and share their input with the therapist and the other group members, the therapist uses descriptive patterning, a graphic organizing tool, to document individual feedback in a large and easy-to-read format for the participants to refer back to as they engage in the different creative arts activities. After a theme has been chosen and discussed, the therapist, using music as a backdrop, then guides the participants through a meditation exercise (step 2, music and meditation). The participants share what memories, thoughts, or feelings came to mind during the meditation, which the therapist adds to the graphic organizing tool. The therapist then leads the group in using what they each saw, felt, or remembered in subsequent creative arts sessions. Chapter 3 offers thematic programming adaptations for people with mild, moderate, or severe Alzheimer's for each step of the TTAP Method, as well as intergenerational uses and adaptations for family members.

Chapter 4 reviews current research related to the physiology of the different regions of the brain and how the brain processes memory. Studies on brain plasticity and the phenomenon of cognitive reserve demonstrate the brain's ability to regain cells lost over time in response to influences and experiences as a person ages, including for those with Alzheimer's. The TTAP Method incorporates this knowledge into an approach that stimulates different regions of the brain in an effort to regrow brain cells and delays the progression of Alzheimer's. The chapter also details current research on Alzheimer's disease, including how depression, emotions, and stress can negatively affect memory and cognitive functioning and the importance of early intervention in treating the disease.

Chapter 5 builds on the discussion of how the TTAP Method stimulates brain functioning by explaining the foundations of the approach in relation to current research on learning and intelligence, specifically Benjamin Bloom's six levels of learning and Howard Gardner's seven learning styles. Readers will better understand how each of the steps of the TTAP Method is designed and structured to stimulate particular types of learners (visual, musical, linguistic, interpersonal, intrapersonal, kinesthetic, and spatial). Understanding that individuals comprehend information differently validates and gives reason to approaching the therapeutic experience using different learning styles, an inherent feature of the TTAP Method. Chapter 5 also discusses the role that emotions, imagination, and creativity play in stimulating the brain and how the TTAP Method integrates each into the creative arts therapeutic experience. The chapter appendix presents a 2009 study of the use of the TTAP Method to stimulate brain functioning in people with moderate to severe Alzheimer's living in a skilled nursing facility.

Chapter 6 begins with a discussion of two distinct areas that are the theoretical underpinnings of the TTAP Method: theories on aging that stress the importance of activities throughout the life span, and the theoretical framework on which therapeutic recreation was founded. Developmental theory and lifespan theory explain why people do what they do and are the theoretical structures out of which the TTAP Method has grown. Having an understanding of the theoretical framework enables the therapist to create a programming structure by which to facilitate for individuals self-determination, self-efficacy, optimal experiences, and a sense of overall well-being. The chapter goes on to discuss several other aging and human development theories that the TTAP Method integrates, including person-centered theory, neurodevelopmental theory, object relations theory, theme-centered interaction theory, and the theory of gerotranscendence. The chapter concludes with a discussion of the evolution of the TTAP Method as a taxonomy, or classification, of learning and cognitive stimulation for people with Alzheimer's disease and other dementias.

Chapter 7 addresses the need for more research on the effectiveness of therapeutic art and recreation for those who have Alzheimer's disease. By creating charts, graphs, and session protocols, the therapist can provide structured documentation with respect to the scope, frequency, and duration of the programming, thereby enhancing the effectiveness of the assessment and evaluation of treatment outcomes. Structured documentation can also assist the therapist in showing how the creative arts programming directly improves a client's treatment outcome, monetarily affects the facility, and increases opportunities for research. The chapter provides examples of documentation of the effectiveness of the TTAP Method as well as sample session protocols from three studies: a 2009 study at a skilled nursing facility at Bergen Regional Medical Center in New Jersey; a 2009 Cornell University study at the Burke Rehabilitation Institute's Memory and Evaluation Clinic in New York; and a 2010 study at Northern Manor Geriatric Center in New York.

The TTAP Method is designed to give the reader a structured and systematic approach for developing creative arts activities to better meet the social, emotional, cognitive, and physical needs of individuals with Alzheimer's disease and other forms of dementia at each stage of the disease progression. This book provides concrete examples of how to perform a guided imagery session, step-by-step examples of thematic sessions, sample protocols to implement, and an activity assessment form to evaluate individual performance and outcomes. The TTAP Method also enables the researching clinician to structure programming and to document what physiological areas are stimulated within the brain, which learning processes are initiated, and the specific length of time the individual is engaged in any given intervention, making this approach consistently replicable to encourage further efficacy research in the field of arts in health care worldwide. Health care providers, caregivers, family members, and professionals can use the TTAP Method to develop multiple creative arts opportunities to engage and revive the mind, body, and spirit of individuals diagnosed with Alzheimer's disease.

CHAPTER 1

Overview of Alzheimer's Disease

Alzheimer's disease is a fatal, degenerative disease of the brain that causes a slow decline in memory, thinking, and reasoning skills. It was first identified by German psychiatrist Alois Alzheimer in 1906. At that time, the beginning of the 20th century, the average life expectancy was 47 years. Most people, therefore, died young enough to avoid this late-life disease. Since then, life expectancy has risen dramatically, from 47 years to 78 years in the United States (Centers for Disease Control and Prevention, 2009). As a result, Alzheimer's has become more prevalent. An estimated 5.4 million Americans of all ages had Alzheimer's disease in 2011, which includes 5.2 million people ages 65 and older and 200,000 individuals under age 65 who have younger-onset Alzheimer's. In 2010, 40 million Americans were more than 65 years old. One in eight of these people had some form of Alzheimer's disease, including 43 percent of people age 85 and older (Alzheimer's Association, 2011). Alzheimer's is the sixth-leading cause of death in the United States, is the most common form of dementia in older adults, and represents more than 70% of all forms of dementia (National Institute on Aging, 2005).

Alzheimer's is a devastating, debilitating neurodegenerative condition that is caused by the deterioration of brain cells. The early stages of the disease are thought to occur at the synapse, since synapse loss is associated with memory dysfunction (University of California–San Diego, 2009). A *synapse* is a structure that permits a nerve cell, or *neuron*, to pass an electrical or chemical signal to another cell. The human brain contains about 10 billion neurons. On average, each neuron is connected to other neurons through about 10,000 synapses. Short outgrowths of *dendrites* (extensions of neurons) relay electrical impulses in the brain (Figure 1.1.A, B). A single neuron's dendrite contains hundreds of thousands of spines, providing memory storage and transmission of signals across synapses. The ability of these spines to change and grow, a process called *plasticity*, is essential for the transmission of signaling in the brain and the support of memory and cognitive functioning (see Chapter 4 for a discussion of brain plasticity and memory).

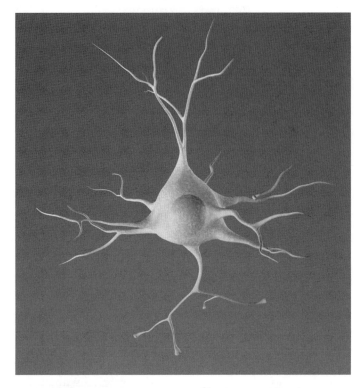

Figure 1.1. (A) Healthy dendrite in a human brain growing from the cell body like healthy roots of a plant.

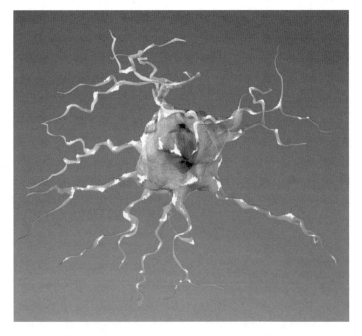

Figure 1.1. (B) Deteriorating dendrite in a human brain affected by Alzheimer's disease. (Images courtesy of the National Institute on Aging/National Institutes of Health, http://www.nia.nih.gov/alzheimers/scientific-images)

Evidence suggests that *beta amyloid* protein plays an important role in the development of Alzheimer's, specifically as a collection of plaques and tangles that accumulate around brain cells. The beta amyloid plaques clump together and attach themselves to neurons in the brain. Once attached, the fibers of plaque prevent the neurons from receiving signals from other cells in the brain. The affected neurons cannot function or communicate with other brain cells, and they die as a result.

The disease typically progresses through three stages: mild, moderate, and severe (Figure 1.2.A, B, C; see Chapter 4). In the first, or mild, stage, a person experiences some memory loss, inability to remember short-term events, and difficulty engaging in prolonged and detailed verbal conversations. In the second, or moderate, stage, the individual shows signs of continued social withdrawal and significant forgetfulness and other cognitive impairment that affects reasoning, self-expression, and the ability to initiate or organize actions. He or she moves from independence to dependence with activities of daily living, specifically bathing, dressing, grooming, eating, toileting, and shopping. By the third, or severe, stage of the disease, a person may experience incontinence, an inability to walk, very serious confusion, loss of speech, and a complete loss of all skills to engage in activities of daily living (Reisberg, de Ferris, Leon, & Crook, 1982).

Alzheimer's disease accounts for an estimated 60% to 80% of all dementia disorders in older adults. In the United States, 100,000 deaths per year are attributed to the disease. In the past 50 years, Alzheimer's has grown from relative obscurity to become a defining characteristic of industrialized society. In 1950, roughly 200,000 Americans were living with the disease. In 2011, the number stood at 5.4 million, including 5.2 million age 65 and older. By 2050, barring discovery of a cure or prevention, from 11 to 16 million Americans are expected to have Alzheimer's, out of a total of 80 million people with the diagnosis worldwide. The disease develops as a result of multiple factors versus a single cause. Prominent risk factors include advancing age, family history, inheriting the ApoE4 gene, mild cognitive impairment (MCI), cardiovascular disease, and head trauma or traumatic brain injury (Alzheimer's Association, 2011).

In addition to memory loss and gradual loss of cognition functioning, as many as 90% of people with Alzheimer's demonstrate clinically significant behavioral and psychological symptoms during the course of the illness, which are believed to be caused in part by a lack of ability to communicate, resulting in severe emotional suffering for those with the disease and often for their caregivers as well. Caring for people with Alzheimer's imposes an immense burden on caregivers because

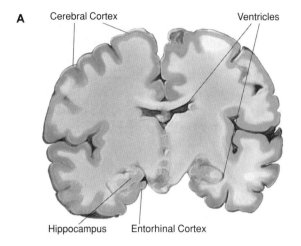

A

Cerebral Cortex   Ventricles

Hippocampus   Entorhinal Cortex

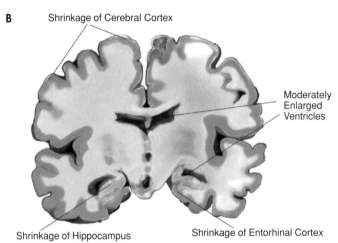

B

Shrinkage of Cerebral Cortex

Moderately
Enlarged
Ventricles

Shrinkage of Hippocampus   Shrinkage of Entorhinal Cortex

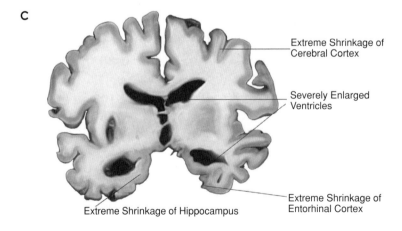

C

Extreme Shrinkage of
Cerebral Cortex

Severely Enlarged
Ventricles

Extreme Shrinkage of Hippocampus

Extreme Shrinkage of
Entorhinal Cortex

Figure 1.2. (A, B, C) Regions of the brain destroyed during the progression of Alzheimer's disease. *A*, preclinical Alzheimer's; *B*, mild to moderate Alzheimer's; and *C*, severe Alzheimer's. (Images courtesy of the National Institute on Aging/ National Institutes of Health, http://www.nia.nih.gov/alzheimers/scientific-images)

they often do not understand what *can* still be done to mentally, physically, and emotionally stimulate the person. More often, the emphasis is on what the person *cannot* do, which can cause great distress for a caregiver who is often left without adequate support or knowledge of ways to stimulate cognitive functioning (Abrisqueta-Gomez et al., 2004).

A definitive diagnosis of Alzheimer's is difficult; confirmation usually can be made only on autopsy. A mental status examination, such as the Folstein Mini–Mental Status Exam, can assess the individual's functional cognitive losses (Folstein, Folstein, & McHugh, 1975). The exam, which lasts about 10 minutes, is composed of 10 short-answer questions that cover orientation to person, place, and time; language abilities; memory recall; and sequencing with fine motor coordination.

As the U.S. population ages, baby boomers (the largest aging cohort) are estimated to increase the number of people with Alzheimer's to more than 10 million by the year 2020. Alzheimer's disease will become an enormous public health problem. Interventions that could delay disease onset even modestly could have a major public health impact (Brookmeyer, Gray, & Kawas, 1998). During a 2008 presentation to the American Society on Aging, the late Gene Cohen announced that if we as a nation could prevent all people from going into a skilled nursing facility, overall health care costs in the United States would decrease by 50%.

WARNING SIGNS OF ALZHEIMER'S DISEASE

Memory loss associated with aging is different from the symptoms of Alzheimer's disease, which increasingly disrupts daily life as cognitive functioning declines. The Alzheimer's Association has developed the following list to help people distinguish the symptoms of the disease from changes in memory that are a part of normal aging. A person may experience one or more of the following common symptoms to different degrees:

- *Memory loss that disrupts daily life.* Forgetting recently learned information or important dates or events. Asking for the same information over and over. Relying on family members or memory aids (written notes or lists) to recall names, tasks, or events. (A typical age-related change is sometimes forgetting a name or an appointment but remembering it later.)

- *Challenges in solving problems or planning.* Decreased ability to develop and follow a plan or work with numbers. Trouble following a familiar recipe or keeping track of monthly bills. Difficulty concentrating. Needing more time than before to accomplish familiar tasks. (A typical age-related change is making occasional errors when balancing a checkbook.)

- *Difficulty completing familiar tasks at home, at work, or at leisure.* Trouble driving to a familiar location, managing a budget at work, or remembering the rules of a favorite game. (A typical age-related change is occasionally needing help to use the settings on a microwave or to record a television show.)

- *Confusion with time or place.* Losing track of dates, seasons, or the passage of time. Difficulty understanding something if it is not happening immediately. Forgetting where one is or how one got there. (A typical age-related change is being confused about the day of the week but figuring it out later.)

- *Trouble understanding visual images and spatial relationships.* Difficulty reading, judging distance, and determining color or contrast. Problems with perception. For example, an individual with Alzheimer's may pass a mirror and think someone else is in the room; the person may not realize it is his or her image that is reflected in the mirror. (A typical age-related change is vision changes related to cataracts.)

- *Problems with language.* Trouble following or joining a conversation, including stopping in the middle of a conversation and having no idea how to continue, or repeating oneself. Problems finding the right word and calling things by the wrong name, such as calling a watch a "hand-clock." (A typical age-related change is sometimes having trouble finding the right word.)

- *Misplacing things and losing the ability to retrace steps.* Putting things in unusual places, such as car keys in the refrigerator. Losing something and being unable to retrace steps to find it again. In some cases (and possibly increasing over time), accusing others of stealing. (A typical age-related change is misplacing things from time to time, such as a pair of glasses or the remote control.)

- *Decreased or poor judgment.* Poor judgment or decision making, such as giving large amounts of money to telemarketers. Being inappropriate or uncharacteristic in grooming or dressing. (A typical age-related change is making a bad decision once in a while.)

- *Withdrawal from work or social activities.* Removing oneself from hobbies, social activities, or work projects. Having trouble keeping up with a favorite sports team or remembering how to engage in a favorite hobby. Possibly, avoiding social interaction because of changes in cognitive abilities. (A typical age-related change is sometimes feeling weary of work, family, and social obligations.)

- *Changes in mood and personality.* Increased feelings of confusion, suspicion, depression, fearfulness, or anxiety. Becoming easily upset at home, at work, with friends, or in places where the person feels out of his or her comfort zone. (A typical age-related change is developing very specific ways of doing things and becoming irritable when a routine is disrupted.)

STAGES OF ALZHEIMER'S DISEASE

As described earlier, the progression of Alzheimer's disease is characterized by three stages: mild (or early), moderate (or mid), and severe (or late). Although the stages can provide a useful framework for understanding how the disease may unfold, not everyone experiences the same symptoms or progresses at the same rate. On average, people with Alzheimer's die 4 to 8 years after diagnosis. Some individuals, however, live as long as 20 years with the disease (Alzheimer's Association, 2011).

The appendix to this chapter outlines the key symptoms of each of the three main stages of Alzheimer's, as well as the other widely used concepts of very mild, moderately severe, and very severe cognitive decline. This stage model is based on a system developed by Dr. Barry Reisberg, clinical director of the New York University School of Medicine's Silberstein Aging and Dementia Research Center. Alternate descriptions of strengths and abilities are included alongside the characterizations of loss and decline associated with each stage. This alternate type of staging, based on strengths and abilities, can be more helpful for care providers and family members in developing individualized care approaches that effectively meet the cognitive, emotional, physical, and social needs of people with Alzheimer's.

A main objective of the Therapeutic Thematic Arts Programming Method (TTAP Method®) is to continually capitalize on the remaining strengths and abilities of people with Alzheimer's through meaningful outlets for self-expression that stimulate all existing areas of brain functioning and the development of alternative cognitive functions to retrieve old memories and enhance old skills. (See Chapter 2 for a more complete discussion of the importance of identifying the existing skills and abilities that a person with Alzheimer's possesses.)

PROGRESSION OF ALZHEIMER'S DISEASE

Mild or Early-Stage Alzheimer's

Identifying the first symptoms of Alzheimer's is crucial for beginning the process of structuring care and treatment. During the early stages of the disease a person experiences loss of memory and cognitive ability that affects daily living. Often people with early-stage Alzheimer's try to hide from others the memory problems they are having. Usually something in the individual's daily habits changes and triggers a family member or caregiver to seek a diagnosis. Difficulties with language (finding the right word) and problems with naming objects are common early warning signs of the disease. These problems can start to occur in social settings, when the person forgets the name or face of someone he or she has known for many years. The function governing language and object names rests in the left side of the brain; scientists still do not know why this side of the brain is the first affected by the abnormal plaques and tangles that cause Alzheimer's.

Moderate or Mid-Stage Alzheimer's

As an individual progresses into the moderate stages of Alzheimer's, a common warning sign is the confusion of place and time as well as a sense of no longer being in control. A person may go for a walk or a drive and suddenly be unable to recall a street name or not know where she is or how she got there. She may need to ask for help to find her way home. Often people with Alzheimer's continue to drive in the moderate stages of the disease process until problems with judgment and orientation become more acute. Problems with memory, concentration, and planning or sequencing also develop during the moderate stage and can affect several daily living skills, such as handling money and paying bills on time. (Chapters 2 and 3 discuss use of the TTAP Method to improve memory and concentration. Chapter 4 discusses the role that positive emotions play in enhancing memory and cognition.)

As the use of language becomes increasingly difficult in the moderate stages of the disease, family members watch a loved one struggle to gather his or her thoughts. A common yet natural mistake is for family members to continue to communicate with the person as they always have in the past. Family members and caregivers need to learn to communicate differently with people with Alzheimer's to effectively engage them. Step 1 of the TTAP Method addresses the importance of communication in meeting the needs of people with Alzheimer's (see Chapter 3).

Severe or Late-Stage Alzheimer's

The loss of cognitive ability to relate appropriately to person, place, and time naturally causes an individual in the severe to late stage of Alzheimer's to verbalize less about his or her needs (Kluger, Ferris, Golomb, Mittelman, & Reisberg, 1999; Levine Madori, 2007). Due to feelings of inadequacy, a person will increasingly refuse to socialize in family gatherings. He or she has a shorter attention span, and judgment becomes increasingly impaired. As a result, the person cannot be left alone, for his or her own well-being and, in some cases, for the well-being of others (the stove might be left on, or the house might be left unlocked). The increasing needs for care and supervision frequently lead to placing the individual in some type of home-care or long-term-care setting, such as assisted living or a skilled nursing facility.

In the last stages of the disease process, assistance with day-to-day activities becomes essential due to severe deficiencies in cognitive functioning. Common behaviors include decreased motor coordination; difficulty sleeping; inability to recall name, address, phone number, or age; increased wandering; refusal to dress or undress; greater assistance needed with activities of daily living; inability to complete simple tasks; use of repetitive sounds or words; being easily overwhelmed by noise or distractions; urinary or fecal incontinence; inability to recognize one's reflection in a mirror; difficulty with balance and walking; and an inability to recognize family and friends.

But even in the late stage of Alzheimer's, people still have abilities. They can respond to music verbally or physically, do simple movements with a colorful balloon, sing the words to a favorite song, look at photo books on topics they enjoy, sort by color or shape, fold small towels and other fabrics, enjoy looking at children or pictures of children, and put things together, such as simple puzzles or blocks.

FAMILY PARTICIPATION AND THE TTAP METHOD

Much of the focus of this book is on the use of the TTAP Method in formal care settings by therapists working with groups of individuals with Alzheimer's; however, the TTAP Method can also be used effectively by family caregivers on a one-to-one basis. With each new discovery about the brain, it becomes increasingly apparent that a person with Alzheimer's needs the support and structure that a family naturally provides. Specifically, the more he or she is spoken to and interacted with, the less rapid the decline in cognitive function (Burgener, Buettner, Beattie, & Rose, 2009; Burgener, Gilbert, & Mathy, 2007; Fratiglioni, Paillard-Borg, & Winblad, 2004). Studies focused on psychosocial interventions have demonstrated that people with mild cognitive impairment, which is cur-

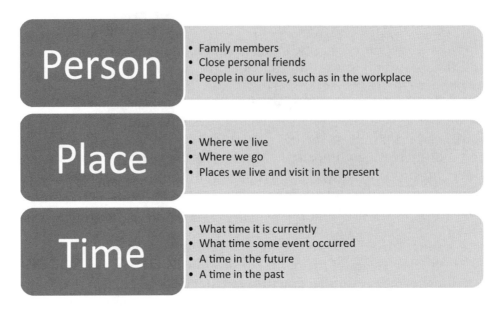

Figure 1.3. How those not diagnosed with Alzheimer's or other dementias commonly communicate (in relation to person, place, and time).

rently recognized as a very early or mild form of Alzheimer's disease, have specific social, emotional, cognitive, and physical needs (Bossen, Specht, & McKenzie, 2009; Davie et al., 2004). Research suggests that activities in the mental, physical, and social domains offer protection against rapid cognitive decline and delay the onset of dementia (Diamond, 2000; Fratiglioni et al., 2004; Kramer et al., 2004). More specifically, continued active participation in social interactions and activities that are individualized and person centered has been shown to enhance feelings of self-esteem and to improve overall quality of life (Gilley, Wilson, Bienias, Bennett, & Evans, 2004; Ostbye, Krause, Norton, Tschanz, & Sanders, 2006; Pruessner, Lord, Meaney, & Lupien, 2004). A national study of all research related to mild or early-stage Alzheimer's concluded that psychosocial support for people newly diagnosed should be in place soon after diagnosis to prevent the self-isolation that can occur as the disease progresses and that can actually accelerate cognitive decline, leading to increased rates of institutionalization (Abrisqueta-Gomez et al., 2004; National Institute on Aging, 2005). Family members can play a very important role in these regards.

The involvement of family provides an important means for people with Alzheimer's to stay connected through words, shared thoughts and memories, and stimulating interactions. How family members communicate with someone with Alzheimer's is vital for the person's overall functioning. Daily and weekly conversations that are structured to stimulate memory and language and to reinforce daily living skills offer the most significant protection in delaying the progression

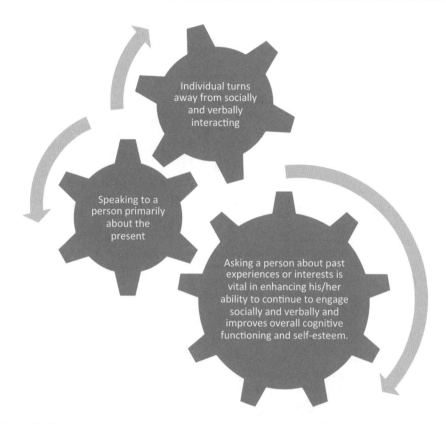

Figure 1.4.   The cycle triggered by the gradual breakdown in communication for people with Alzheimer's.

of the disease and can also improve cognitive functioning (Bottino, Carvalho, & Alvarez, 2002; Burgener et al., 2007; Zanetti et al., 1997).

An individual with Alzheimer's gradually loses the ability to communicate, creating a cycle of frustration and distress for the person as well as for his or her family members (Figure 1.3), in part because family members continue trying to communicate with a loved one as they always have in the past. We learn how to socialize and structure conversation in relation to person, place, or time. We speak about *people* in our lives whom we know. We speak about *places* we occupy or visit (home, office, shop, concert hall, beach). We speak about *times* we have experienced, whether in reference to the current day, a date in the future, or an event that occurred in the past. As the disease progresses, the individual loses the ability to communicate in relation to person, place, and time. When a family member naturally tries to communicate with the loved one, it becomes increasingly stressful and frustrating for both; the family member is looking for a response, and the individual with Alzheimer's cannot give one. This gradual breakdown in communication triggers a cycle of self-isolation on the part of a person with Alzheimer's, as well as mounting frustration and resentment on the part of the family member (Figure 1.4).

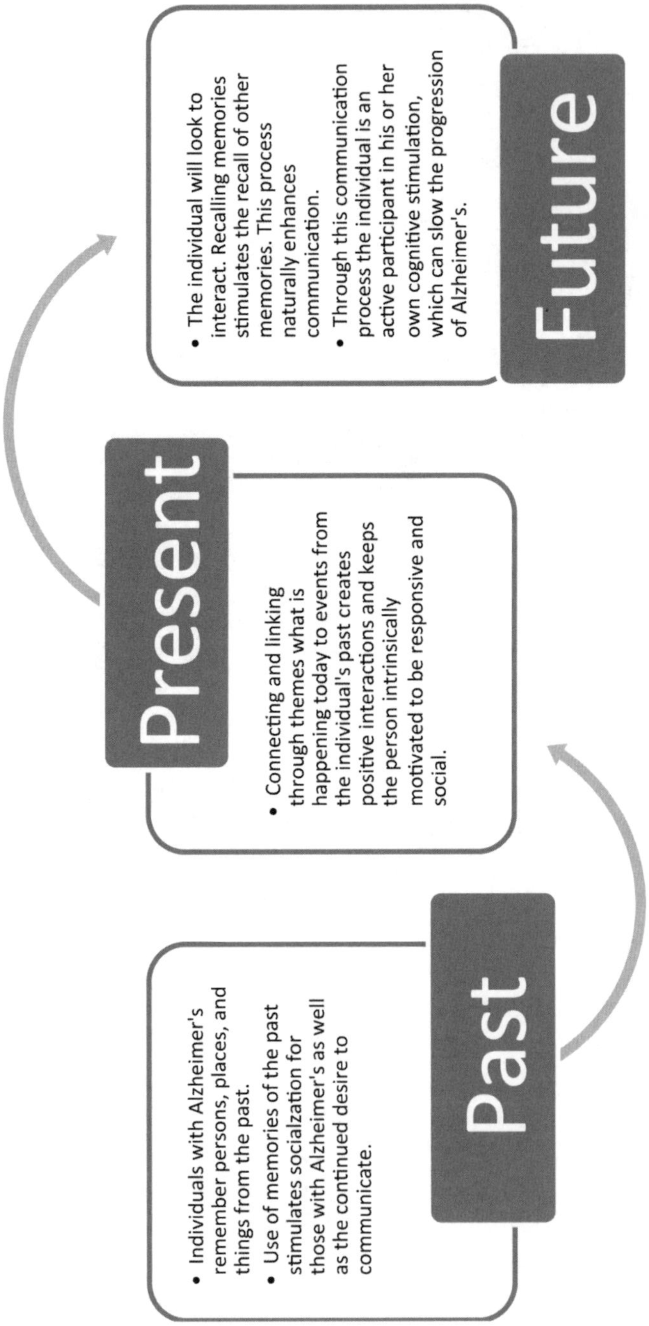

Figure 1.5.   Communication through the TTAP Method.

Past

- Individuals with Alzheimer's remember persons, places, and things from the past.
- Use of memories of the past stimulates socialzation for those with Alzheimer's as well as the continued desire to communicate.

Present

- Connecting and linking through themes what is happening today to events from the individual's past creates positive interactions and keeps the person intrinsically motivated to be responsive and social.

Future

- The individual will look to interact. Recalling memories stimulates the recall of other memories. This process naturally enhances communication.
- Through this communication process the individual is an active participant in his or her own cognitive stimulation, which can slow the progression of Alzheimer's.

Family members can use the TTAP Method to improve communication with their loved one. Long-term memories stay with a person who has Alzheimer's well into the disease process. Communication using the TTAP Method stimulates the recall of long-term memories. Figure 1.5 illustrates the communication process using the TTAP Method, specifically using themes to connect to the individual's past, which increases the quality of interactions and verbal responsiveness, which in turn decreases the risk of self-isolation. Chapters 2 and 3 discuss communication through the TTAP Method, including how family members can use past memories tied to objects found in every home to stimulate rich interactions, responsiveness, and verbalizations.

CONCLUSION

Researchers continue to make advances in diagnosing Alzheimer's disease and other dementias as well as identifying potential risk factors. To date, however, there is no cure or effective treatment for Alzheimer's. Brain research has revealed that continual stimulation of memory, both short and long term, plays an integral role in the wellness of the brain and, thus, in overall quality of life. Research is also demonstrating a high correlation between creative processes and decreased heart rate, increased activity in specific areas of the brain, and an overall improved sense of self and well-being. Family and professional caregivers have a growing number of care approaches centered around activities programming that have proven successful in engaging those with Alzheimer's, even into the later stages.

This book is intended to bring a growing body of knowledge to the field of creative arts therapy to assist therapists in better assessing, implementing, developing, planning, and evaluating the therapeutic process by using the TTAP Method for those with Alzheimer's and other dementias. It is recommended for the professional therapist who is teaching or practicing; for the instructor who is teaching in creative arts therapy; for the student in creative arts therapy and therapeutic recreation; and for the sibling, spouse, child, or friend who needs direction with what to do with an older person who has some form of dementia. The TTAP Method is designed specifically for therapists who work with the largest special group ever to exist: older adults. The more that therapists understand about the physiological, psychological, and social needs of individuals with Alzheimer's, the better they can provide therapeutic recreation through the use of creative arts therapies.

Stages of Alzheimer's Disease: An Alternative Perspective

Loss/Decline	Strengths/Abilities
Stage 1: No impairment Normal function	
• Unimpaired individuals experience no memory problems and none are evident to a health care professional during a medical interview.	• Fully functioning person
Stage 2: Very mild cognitive decline May be normal age-related changes or earliest signs of Alzheimer's disease	
• Individuals may feel as if they have memory lapses, especially in forgetting familiar words or names or the location of keys, eyeglasses, or other everyday objects. But these problems are not evident during a medical examination or apparent to friends, family, or co-workers.	• Fully functioning person who may forget something from time to time.
Stage 3: Mild cognitive decline Early-stage Alzheimer's can be diagnosed in some, but not all, individuals with these symptoms.	
Friends, family, or co-workers begin to notice deficiencies. Problems with memory or concentration may be measurable in clinical testing or discernible during a detailed medical interview. Common difficulties include the following:	A person remains able to do the following:
• Word- or name-finding problems noticeable to family or close associates	• Engage in conversations with others although may need support with some words
• Decreased ability to remember names when introduced to new people • Performance issues in social or work settings noticeable to family, friends, or co-workers	• Meet new people and socialize although may not be able to refer to them by name all the time
• Reading a passage and retaining little material	• Enjoy reading short passages and stories
• Losing or misplacing a valuable object	• Locate misplaced items with help
• Decline in ability to plan or organize	• Plan uncomplicated tasks and activities or more complicated tasks with support and assistance

Loss/Decline	Strengths/Abilities
Stage 4: Moderate cognitive decline Mild or early-stage Alzheimer's disease	
At this stage, a careful medical interview detects clear-cut deficiencies in the following areas: • Decreased knowledge of recent occasions or current events	A person remains able to do the following: • Talk about the past in great detail
• Impaired ability to perform challenging mental arithmetic—for example, to count backward from 100 by 7s	• Perform basic arithmetic
• Decreased capacity to perform complex tasks, such as shopping, planning dinner for guests, or paying bills and managing finances	• Perform noncomplex tasks or more complex tasks with assistance
• Reduced memory of personal history	• Recall personal history with reminders or cues
• Increased withdrawal and subdued behavior, especially in socially or mentally challenging situations	• Engage in social and mentally challenging situations when included appropriately or in a simplified manner
Stage 5: Moderately severe cognitive decline Moderate or mid-stage Alzheimer's disease	
Major gaps in memory and deficits in cognitive function emerge. Some assistance with day-to-day activities becomes essential. At this stage, individuals may do the following: • Be unable during a medical interview to recall such important details as their current address, their telephone number, or the name of the college or high school from which they graduated	At this stage, individuals can do the following: • Convey feelings
• Become confused about where they are or about the date, day of the week, or season	• Be in and enjoy the moment
• Have trouble with less challenging mental arithmetic; for example, counting backward from 40 by 4s or from 20 by 2s	• Perform simple mental arithmetic
• Need help choosing proper clothing for the season or the occasion	• Select clothing with limited choices
• Retain substantial knowledge about themselves and know their own name and the names of their spouse or children	• Have knowledge about themselves and know names of spouse and children
• Require no assistance with eating or using the toilet	• Eat and use bathroom independently

(continued)

Loss/Decline	Strengths/Abilities

Stage 6: Severe cognitive decline
Moderately severe or mid-stage Alzheimer's disease

Loss/Decline	Strengths/Abilities
Memory difficulties continue to worsen, significant personality changes may emerge, and affected individuals need extensive help with customary daily activities. At this stage, individuals may do the following:	At this stage, individuals can do the following:
• Lose most awareness of recent experiences and events, as well as of their surroundings	• Talk about past experiences in some detail
• Recollect their personal history imperfectly, although they generally recall their own name	• Know their name and recall personal history with cues
• Occasionally forget the name of their spouse or primary caregiver but generally can distinguish familiar from unfamiliar faces	• Recognize familiar faces and individuals
• Need help getting dressed properly; without supervision, may make such errors as putting pajamas over daytime clothes or shoes on wrong feet	• Dress self with limited choices and support or assistance
• Experience disruption of their normal sleep/waking cycle	• Enjoy an afternoon nap or early morning sunrise
• Need help with handling details of toileting (flushing toilet, wiping and disposing of tissue properly)	• Use the bathroom with cues and support/assistance
• Have increasing episodes of urinary or fecal incontinence	• Use toilet and be successful with reminders
• Experience significant personality changes and behavioral symptoms, including suspiciousness and delusions (for example, believing that their caregiver is an impostor); hallucinations (seeing or hearing things that are not really there); or compulsive, repetitive behaviors such as hand-wringing or tissue shredding	• Perform or assist with tasks that are repetitive in nature
• Tend to wander and become lost	• Move around and take walks with supervision

Loss/Decline	Strengths/Abilities

Stage 7: Very severe cognitive decline
Severe or late-stage Alzheimer's disease

Loss/Decline	Strengths/Abilities
This is the final stage of the disease when individuals lose the ability to respond to their environment, the ability to speak, and, ultimately, the ability to control movement. At this stage, individuals may do the following:	At this stage, individuals can do the following:
• Frequently lose their capacity for recognizable speech, although words or phrases may occasionally be uttered	• Use simple words or phrases and respond nonverbally or with groans
• Need help with eating and toileting and have general incontinence of urine	• Eat with assistance and use the bathroom with assistance
• Lose the ability to walk without assistance, then the ability to sit without support, the ability to smile, and the ability to hold their head up; reflexes become abnormal and muscles grow rigid; swallowing is impaired.	• Walk with help and sit with support • Enjoy tastes of certain flavors

Reprinted with permission from *The Enduring Self in People with Alzheimer's: Getting to the Heart of Individualized Care*, by Sam Fazio (pp. 53–56). Baltimore: Health Professions Press, 2008.

CHAPTER 2

Overview of the Therapeutic Thematic Arts Programming Method

The Therapeutic Thematic Arts Programming Method (TTAP Method®; pronounced TAP) combines the principles of therapeutic recreation and creative arts therapies into a single, structured technique that stimulates different areas of the brain through all creative arts forms, linking each project to a specific brain function. It is an innovative psychological approach that has been proven to positively affect the emotional, social, physical, and cognitive functions of people diagnosed with Alzheimer's disease or other forms of dementia (Alders, 2008; Alders & Levine Madori, 2010; Levine Madori, 2007, 2009a,b,c).

The TTAP Method has grown out of neuroscience research that demonstrates that life experiences (life review, the life story), coupled with activities that challenge the mind, stimulate positive changes in the brain and holistically improve the well-being of an individual (Bohlmeijer, Valenkamp, Westerhof, Smi, & Cuijpers, 2005; Buckwalter, Burgener, & Buettner, 2008; Cohen, 2006; McKenzie, 1996). With rising numbers of people diagnosed with Alzheimer's disease (see Chapter 1), the need is growing for family and professional caregivers, as well as the U.S. health care system generally, to develop and tailor strength-based interventions to promote the retention of skills and abilities of people across all stages of the disease process (Burgener, Gilbert, & Mathy, 2007; Clare, Wilson, Carter, Roth, & Hodges, 2002; Rentz, 2002).

The need for continual and challenging cognitive stimulation to maintain cognitive functioning has been well documented. By keeping people stimulated for longer periods of time in person-centered art and recreation activities, the TTAP Method naturally encourages intrinsic motivation, thereby increasing feelings of self-esteem, which directly affects the mental, physical, and psychological domains of the individual. (Chapter 5 discusses how the TTAP Method incorporates and stimulates regions of the brain and how continual brain stimulation promotes the creation of new brain cells and the retention of remaining skills and abilities of people with Alzheimer's disease.)

WHAT IS THE TTAP METHOD?

The TTAP Method is a program of activities that revolve around a particular theme over an extended period and that provide a range of therapeutic benefits through two avenues: (1) the expressive arts, including language and communication, meditation, music, dance, and drama, and (2) the physiological effects on the brain promoted by stimulating different regions through varying activities. By incorporating all seven learning styles (linguistic, logical, spatial, musical, kinesthetic, interpersonal, and intrapersonal), the TTAP Method offers opportunities for success in areas of individual strength, which promotes feelings of inclusion and efficacy for each participant during all structured steps of the activity. (See Chapter 5 for a full discussion of Howard Gardner's seven learning styles and how the TTAP Method incorporates them.)

The TTAP Method has six main objectives:

1. To stimulate all areas of brain functioning to enhance cognitive, emotional, physical, and social capacity.

2. To provide opportunities for the individual to integrate life experiences into group experiences that tie the creative arts process to a theme, object, or prop.

3. To provide a system in which the individual can reintegrate into a supportive social group to foster feelings of safety and support and thereby increase social participation.

4. To engage the participant in multiple creative arts experiences, including music, drawing, sculpture, movement, poetry, and special theme events.

5. To provide programming that enables the experience of a state of *flow*, the concept of being in the "optimal experience," which contributes to the emotional, psychological, social, and physical wellness of the individual (see discussion later in this chapter).

6. To enhance communication in all care settings, including community services for well elderly, rehabilitation programs, assisted living facilities, skilled nursing care, and services for Alzheimer's disease (Levine Madori, 2007).

THE VALUE OF THEMES

The use of themes in the TTAP Method is essential. A theme provides a focus for exploring all areas of a single topic. Thematic programming is a process that facilitates creative thinking, then brainstorming, and finally implementation. The TTAP Method provides the therapist with the structure to explore a theme, from which group participants can take off in multiple directions using creative arts therapy. The input of each person in a group is significant; thematic programming gives each person an opportunity to express individual thinking and promotes interaction with others and the sharing of self, each maximizing self-esteem.

The TTAP Method has benefits for the therapist as well as for the participant. Thinking in a thematic way allows the therapist to incorporate his or her own experiences while also sharing ideas from the group. It keeps the therapeutic programming innovative and fresh. Themes provide a natural way of learning and processing information through activities. Another beauty of theme subjects is that they are broad; they allow open-ended brainstorming to take place in a structured yet flexible environment.

Thematic programming provides the following benefits:

- Themes provide a natural way of learning and processing information through activities.

- Thematic programming lets participants form a deep understanding of or relationship with the subject or topic.

- Thematic programming is structured yet flexible and allows for individualization that meets clients' learning needs or stimulates interests that already have been cultivated.

- Thematic programming is a vehicle through which all creative arts therapies can be involved, complementing the therapeutic process and enriching the therapeutic outcome.

- Thematic programming can establish creative activities that flow together rather than being isolated events whose benefits fail to carry over into everyday aspects of care.

- Theme subjects are broad; they allow open-ended brainstorming to take place yet provide some structure and direction for participants.

- Themes have significant relevance to real life.

The thematic programming process has three main goals:

1. To use creative expression to reveal a fundamental link between each person's self-esteem and intrinsic motivation and to encourage this process to take place continually within the group

2. To continually draw on past and present personal pursuits, life experiences, and interests that have accrued across the life span to elevate each person's self-expression to a central position in all programming

3. To recognize and continually support each person's unique combination of skills, multiple intelligences, and capabilities for self-expression

These goals are accomplished by using connected creative activities around a theme to provide a stimulating and rich group experience for the participants.

STEPS OF THE TTAP METHOD

Each TTAP Method program begins with the therapist guiding the group in conversation about a chosen theme (step 1). The therapist next leads the group through a music and meditation exercise (step 2), to relax the participants as well as focus them on the activity theme. The group is then engaged in a creative arts activity (painting and drawing, phototherapy, movement and dance, etc. [steps 3–11]). The order in which steps 3 through 11 are outlined and discussed in this book need not be followed literally; the steps can be changed to suit the needs of the participants, and they can be repeated as often as the participants desire. Each TTAP Method program ends with the therapist gathering client feedback to use in assessing the effectiveness of the programming (step 12).

Step 1: From individual thought to group conversation

Step 2: From group conversation to music and meditation

Step 3: From music and meditation to drawing and painting

Step 4: From drawing and painting to sculpture

Step 5: From sculpture to movement and dance

Step 6: From movement and dance to personal or group writing experience (poetry, stories)

Step 7: From personal or group writing experience to food experience

Step 8: From food experience to theme event

Step 9: From theme event to phototherapy

Step 10: From phototherapy to sensory stimulation

Step 11: From sensory stimulation to drama or theater experience

Step 12: Client feedback, assessment, and evaluation

(Chapter 3 discusses in detail each step and gives examples of how to apply the TTAP Method to people with dementia. Chapters 3 and 5 identify which parts of the brain each step stimulates and how.)

THE CCDERS APPROACH™ AND THE TTAP METHOD

The TTAP Method incorporates and promotes six often overlooked but common strengths and abilities that a person with Alzheimer's possesses throughout the disease process. These include the ability and desire to

> *Communicate* with others
>
> *Connect* with others
>
> *Differentiate* likes and dislikes
>
> *Express* feelings and emotions
>
> *Recall* long-term memories
>
> *Self-express* pleasurable emotions and receiving joy

I developed the CCDERS Approach™ based in part on the work of Tabourne and McKenzie, who have shown the importance of life review and reminiscence therapy for people diagnosed with Alzheimer's (discussed in Chapter 6). These abilities can be understood more fully as follows:

> *Communicate with others:* People with Alzheimer's do not lose the desire to communicate simply because the disease causes them to have difficulty expressing themselves. They want to communicate, and they continue to have the desire to do so, specifically with others through a group experience.
>
> *Connect with others:* As people age, their circle of social relationships can shrink, yet the desire for social connections does not lessen. A person with Alzheimer's has the same desire to connect with others as the person who ages normally. The group experience that is created by the TTAP Method naturally allows this to occur.
>
> *Differentiate likes and dislikes:* People diagnosed with Alzheimer's can and still want to differentiate themselves through their personal preferences. They still have the ability to favor one

color over another, for example. They still want to retain personhood and the ability to express who they are, what they like, and what they do not like.

Express feelings and emotions: Through the slow cognitive decline of dementia, the use of words and language starts to fade, but the person can still express feelings and emotions. The expression often occurs through body language; for example, a person says "I" and hugs herself to communicate "I love you."

Recall long-term memories: The first significant loss in the Alzheimer's disease process is short-term memory. However, a person with Alzheimer's still has the functioning mental capacity to recall long-term memories, specifically memories that have strong emotional meaning to the person. Speaking about themes is a natural way to evoke personal memories so that they can be shared through the recall process.

Self-express pleasurable emotions and receiving joy: All people, even those diagnosed with Alzheimer's, want to engage in self-expression by sharing what they think and feel. The group experience increases the participants' ability to continue to share his or her personal perspective on all themes discussed throughout programming. (See Figure 2.1.)

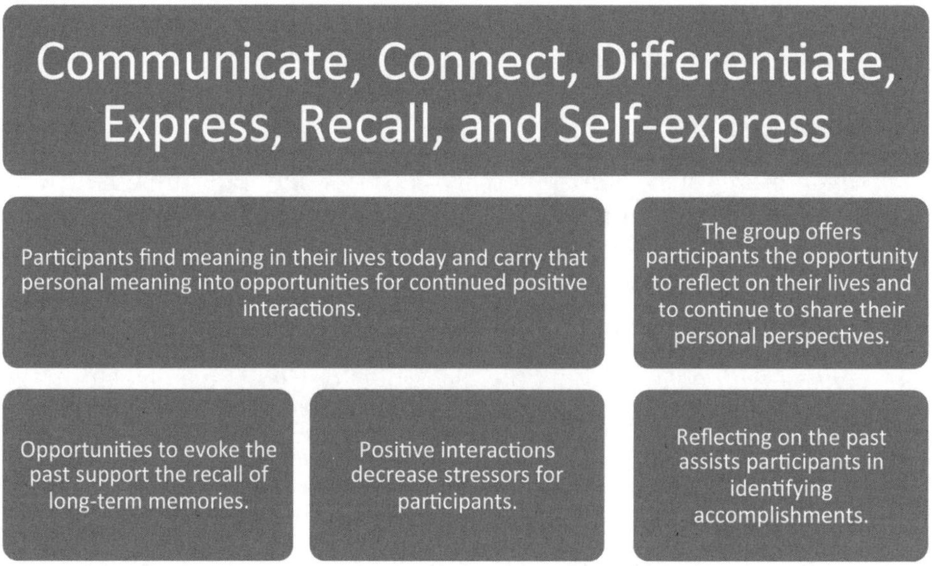

Communicate, Connect, Differentiate, Express, Recall, and Self-express

Participants find meaning in their lives today and carry that personal meaning into opportunities for continued positive interactions.	The group offers participants the opportunity to reflect on their lives and to continue to share their personal perspectives.
Opportunities to evoke the past support the recall of long-term memories.	Positive interactions decrease stressors for participants.
	Reflecting on the past assists participants in identifying accomplishments.

Figure 2.1. The CCDERS Approach incorporates as part of a group experience each of the six common remaining strengths and abilities of individuals with Alzheimer's.

The TTAP Method supports the six common remaining strengths by creating multiple opportunities for life review through the use of a theme or object. (See Chapter 6 for a discussion of object relations theory as it relates to the Alzheimer's population.) For example, an object can be used to draw the focus of an individual with Alzheimer's onto the meaning that the object holds for him or her. This activity stimulates *communication* (the first step of the TTAP Method). Through the ability to be engaged by the object, the person is *connecting* (with the therapist and others in the group). Furthermore, this activity gives group members continual opportunities to express and thus *differentiate* their likes and dislikes related to the object. For instance, if the therapist uses a seashell as part of a themed conversation, the person's ability to reveal his or her likes and dislikes of summers spent on the beach naturally emerges. This closely corresponds to the opportunities the person has to share and *express emotions* related to the object. Long-term memory is not affected by Alzheimer's disease until the later stage. Thus the more opportunities a person with Alzheimer's has to *recall* long-term memories, the better. As conversations and connections are repeated using various objects and themes, the person with Alzheimer's has many opportunities for *self-expression* that the therapist can reinforce by giving repeated positive feedback.

Using the TTAP Method, the therapist or activity professional can develop and assess daily, weekly, or monthly programming interactions to stimulate these six common strengths, drawn primarily from the person's past interests. This holistic psychological approach will guide the therapist or activity professional in finding ways to reintroduce past interests in a dynamic multimodal structure. (See Figure 2.2.) (See Chapter 6 for a discussion of the CCDERS Approach in relation to the Levine Madori Taxonomy.)

APPLYING THE CONCEPTS OF THE TTAP METHOD

The TTAP Method focuses on a single topic while allowing the therapeutic process to unfold within the group experience. In selecting each activity for this process, it is important to consider the participant's skill level and the activity challenge. When the participant's skill level is low and the activity challenge is high, he or she is likely to experience frustration and anxiety. When the skill level and activity challenge are equal, however, the participant is able to achieve a state of concentration and energy expenditure that Csikszentmihalyi (1990) called *flow* (discussed later in this chapter). Participants can achieve flow through the personal choice, self-determination, and self-efficacy that are essential components of the TTAP Method.

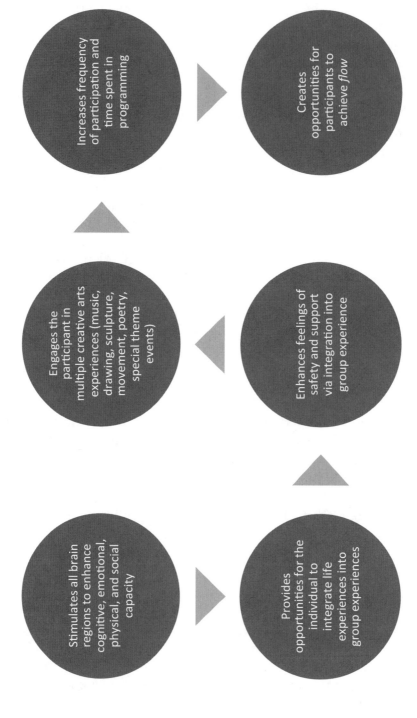

Figure 2.2.   Goals and objectives of the TTAP Method.

TTAP Method Promotes Perceived Freedom Through Personal Choice

In the TTAP Method, participants provide continual input from their personal life experiences, which the therapist incorporates into the group programming. One fundamental concept of leisure behavior is *perceived freedom* (Iso-Ahola, 1980; Mannell & Kleiber, 1997). Perceived freedom means that the activity or behavior in which the person participates is purely for leisure's sake (i.e., actions are chosen freely), not because someone else is forcing participation. The therapist continually solicits input from the participants through conversation and art experiences, thereby fostering participants' free will in choosing to participate and the extent to which they contribute. As research has shown, older adults express the continued need to participate, and that participation, at whatever skill level, is crucial to well-being and quality of life (Levine Madori, 2004).

The role of therapeutic art and recreation is to provide many opportunities for the participant to make personal choices and thereby remain involved in meaningful activities. Among the psychological benefits of the TTAP Method is the opportunity for the participants to believe that they are in control of and contributing to events and activities.

TTAP Method Promotes Intrinsic Motivation Through Self-Determination

Activities that people feel successful performing also allow for the development of self through self-expression and self-awareness. Deci (1975) and Deci and Ryan (1985) first presented the concept of intrinsic motivation as an essential component of the human experience. Mannell and Kleiber (1997) applied the theory of intrinsic motivation to leisure behavior, emphasizing the relationship between freedom of choice and self-determination. People are intrinsically motivated by how something makes them feel. These feelings include personal enjoyment, satisfaction, and gratification. The TTAP Method is structured around each person in the group in a way that allows each group member to receive positive feedback and affirmation from not only the therapist but also other participants, thereby fostering continued feelings of gratification and personal enjoyment. The TTAP Method relies on this constant positive outcome to strengthen the intrinsic motivation to participate.

TTAP Method Promotes Self-Efficacy

Self-efficacy, or competence, is the belief that individuals can exercise control over their own functions and over environmental events to reach a desired end (Bandura, 1997, 2001; Warr, 1993). Efficacy beliefs play an important role in leisure behaviors and leisure pursuits. These beliefs of competence can influence whether the person thinks optimistically or pessimistically, thereby affecting self-enhancing or self-hindering thoughts and behaviors. According to Stumbo and Peterson,

> Efficacy beliefs are fundamental to the individual's sense of competence and control. Individuals with higher self-efficacy believe their choices and actions will affect the outcome of a situation; those with lower self-efficacy believe their choices and actions have little relationship to the outcome. (2004, p. 21)

Bandura (1997) explained that information sources for self-efficacy include (1) vicarious experience (i.e., observing someone else perform a similar task), (2) performance accomplishments (i.e., succeeding at the same or a similar task), (3) verbal persuasion (e.g., "you are able to do this task"), and (4) physiological arousal (i.e., the physical body is ready to perform). The TTAP Method allows each participant to watch as other group members share ideas, interests, and feelings, which offers verbal persuasion not only from the therapist but also—and most important—from peers.

TTAP Method Promotes Optimal Experience

Csikszentmihalyi (1990) popularized the term *flow* for the concept of being in the optimal experience. For a person to achieve flow, a number of elements must be present (Csikszentmihalyi, 1990; Edgington et al., 1998; Heywood, 1978; Mannell & Kleiber, 1997):

- Intense involvement
- Clarity of goals and feedback
- Deep concentration and focus
- Transcendence of self
- Loss of self-consciousness
- Loss of time
- Direct and immediate feedback
- Intrinsically rewarding experience
- Balance between ability level or skill and challenge
- Sense of personal control

Csikszentmihalyi summed up the importance of these elements as follows: "In the long run optimal experiences add up to a sense of mastery—or perhaps better, a sense of *participation* in determining the content of life—that comes as close to what is usually meant by happiness as anything else we can conceivably imagine" (1990, p. 4). The optimal experience contributes to the emotional, psychological, social, and physical wellness of the individual. The TTAP Method offers each of the elements of flow:

- *Intense involvement:* The person discovers multiple forms of art and creative self-expression, creating opportunities for complete absorption into an activity and stimulation of the brain through cognitive challenges.

- *Clarity of goals and feedback:* The structure of the themed programming focuses the person's attention.

- *Deep concentration and focus:* Structure heightens the ability to concentrate and focus.

- *Loss of self-consciousness:* Each step can be adapted to meet the specific needs of the individual, creating a greater sense of self-esteem and satisfaction.

- *Loss of time:* Engaging each participant in the themed activities helps him or her focus intently and in a way that makes the sense of time and place irrelevant.

- *Direct and immediate feedback:* The therapist is able to give repetitive positive feedback for each step and at each stage of the process.

- *Intrinsically rewarding experience:* The person has multiple opportunities for success, whether it is socially rewarding, artistically fulfilling, or verbally satisfying, thus creating intrinsic motivation to continue to engage in the activities.

- *Balance between ability level or skill and challenge:* People of varying skill levels and cognitive abilities can work on a themed activity, thus enabling the therapist to engage participants at all levels of functioning.

- *Sense of personal control:* Each individual is encouraged to bring to an activity something significant from his or her life story, memories, or personal interests. At all times, participants are in control of what they want to do, unlike in traditional art and recreation programs that are less person centered.

By giving the participant the opportunity to revisit a theme continually, the creative arts experience can be extremely rewarding and can ultimately reinforce the flow throughout the experience. This *flow effect* provides structure for each participant and allows the programs to be expanded on; a typical 45-minute session can be increased to an hour and a half. Each participant works on a personal experience while supporting the group. Increased verbalization occurs naturally because the person is being asked to share thoughts that are introspective and relevant and that hold significant meaning. The flow effect will occur during each phase of the programs. Using thematic programming, the therapist can develop and implement activities in the arts, language, and music that all link together around a particular theme.

Music as Therapy in the TTAP Method

Music is an excellent therapy in thematic programming. The mind and the cells of the temporal lobe create a snapshot of emotional events, and these are deeply embedded in the sounds of music. Music activates a flow of stored memories across the brain; as a result, the recall of long-term memories is greatly enhanced. A good example of this phenomenon is hearing a special song on the radio. While driving to your job, picking up the kids, or running errands, you hear a song and suddenly are back in the moment when you first heard the song. That moment could have been last week or 5, 10, or 30 years ago, but all the memories of the people, the place, and the events associated with the song are alive in your mind as if it were only yesterday. The experience of music for someone who has lived a long time is thus extremely beneficial.

Scientists and physicians have been intrigued by the effects that music and movement can have on the brain. Since the mid-1990s, neurological research has been finding that music and movement can be extremely useful in cases of traumatic brain injury, severe autism, profound mental retardation, and end-stage dementia, yet the effects that music has on the brain and functioning are not fully understood. Increasingly, the benefits of music therapy in meeting the social and emotional needs of older adults as well as people with Alzheimer's disease are being researched. Bright (1988) studied music and memory, and particularly how music and dance can stimulate memories in long-term storage when stimuli such as verbal conversation can fail. The response to music occurs through brain mechanisms that are involved in the perception and processing of information. Music can stimulate memories that are still retained in the long-term memory of people with Alzheimer's, whose short-term memory progressively erodes as a result of the disease process.

In clinical studies using music in association with Parkinson's disease, Selman (1988) found that music was vital in helping people with the disease to speak, and participants were able to express a larger range of emotion. The music also assisted in the formation of language through sounds. This stimulation in turn allows new brain pathways to grow and connect, which is essential in slowing the progression of dementia and maintaining cognitive functioning.

The work of providing structures and techniques for self-expression and creativity for the aging person is extremely significant on many different levels. The general objective of music therapy is to give all participants the opportunity for communication and socialization. Music therapy also provides the opportunity for a new means of non-verbal communication. This is especially valuable for the older partici-pant, who may be more isolated or who may have speech limitations. Ultimately, the effectiveness of music therapy is based on two basic components: (1) it stimulates emotions through dramatization while providing safety and emotional reassurance and (2) it opens up new communication channels. The evocative value of music can be used to revive and arouse an emotional world in people with dementia that otherwise may be unexplored or lost entirely as the effects of the dis-ease worsen.

Words as Therapy in the TTAP Method

Using words comes naturally but often is left out of the creative arts. In the course of growing up, people learn how to communicate tales of knowledge, experience, or bewilderment. These stories slowly but steadily become the memories that reflect a person's life. In time, sto-ries that are in short-term memory move into deep storage in long-term memory, where they dwell in embodied silence (Rubin, 1995). The architecture of the memory system is still being discovered and is still a source of wonder. What is certain is that telling personal stories is fundamental to the human experience (Williams & Hollan, 1981); the converse, not telling personal stories, has been proved to have adverse consequences to health. Dr. Ron Kennedy stated, "Nothing can be more important for your health then the unimpeded expression of emotion. Unfortunately, this is not something our culture promotes. The result is that unexpressed emotions express their energy in the living systems of the body, frequently disrupting those systems" (Ken-nedy, 2006, p. 1).

Life experience and research confirm the intuitive sense that a per-sistent inability to tell one's story to relevant people at relevant moments becomes a problem eventually (Donovan, 1996). Stories convey a per-son's knowledge, and telling these stories is simply good for a person.

The capacity to develop through learning is closely related to curi-osity and can be defined as a desire to find an explanation, an interpretation, or something that is of interest. Therapeutic storytelling, poetry, and creative writing support this vital process of constructive exploration in three ways:

- By arousing interest and past memories in events and people that might have been forgotten

- By providing satisfaction with explication and feedback and continuing the exploratory process

- By providing ways to initiate, use, and develop interpersonal relationships

These are the curiosity-supporting functions that are fundamental to the use of creative writing and storytelling; therefore, writing is an essential element in the creative arts experience, especially for older adults with dementia.

Photographs as Therapy in the TTAP Method

Butler (1963) originated the concept of life review using photographs and verbal sharing to revive experiences and survey and reintegrate unresolved conflicts. Life review is the process by which a person comes to terms with the totality of his or her life experiences and fashions a new meaning of the self, which is essential for mental health. (See Chapter 6 for a more detailed discussion of life review as a theoretical underpinning of the TTAP Method.)

People commonly photograph significant events, including births of children, birthdays, weddings, holidays, vacations, and significant people and places in their life. Photographs elicit between people a common bond that can be expressed either verbally or nonverbally.

Weiss and Kronberg (1986) described how nursing assistants for people with Alzheimer's disease encouraged reminiscing by using old photographs. Austin (1995) identified enhanced self-esteem, socialization, stimulated cognition, and expression of feelings as therapeutic benefits of life review. Phototherapy, or the use of reminiscence and photographic images, can have a profound effect on the pleasure centers of the brain (McClellan, 2001). An overall sense of well-being can be achieved through the use of photographic images, whether printed, projected, or viewed as a film.

MULTIMODAL CARE APPROACHES FOR PEOPLE WITH ALZHEIMER'S DISEASE

Various psychological approaches are effective in maintaining and maximizing functioning of people with Alzheimer's disease. The most efficacious approaches have been based on a combination of individualized, interdisciplinary, and holistic treatments. Such multimodal treatment approaches are especially well suited for people experiencing dementia, a progressive disorder. Through the repetitive stimulation of all brain regions through a variety of activities, people with Alzheimer's can actively engage in purposeful and successful activity throughout the disease process (Schindler & Cucio, 2000).

As discussed in Chapter 1, research has shown that activities in the mental, physical, and social domains have protective effects against cognitive decline and dementia (Fratiglioni et al., 2004). More specifically, continued active participation in social interactions and activities that are individualized and person centered enhance feelings of self-esteem and directly improve overall quality of life (Pruessner et al., 2004). The most significant findings have been shown through the use of multimodal care approaches.

THE TTAP METHOD AS A MULTIMODAL APPROACH

Multimodal interventions (a mix of interventions, stimulating all regions of the brain) have proven extremely successful in delaying the disease progression in early-stage Alzheimer's and are designed to provide a wide array of stimuli, affecting neuronal activity and responses through a variety of mechanisms. Rentz (2002) described the use of a variety of art programs through the Memories in the Making® program with mild- to moderate-stage Alzheimer's in an adult day program ($N = 41$). Outcomes included increased well-being, self-esteem, and improved quality of life. Teri and colleagues (2003) conducted a multimodal intervention using exercise and support groups to improve memory and reduce depression ($N = 140$). Post-intervention outcomes included improvement in depression and physical functioning. Most significantly, outcomes were maintained at the 2-year post-intervention evaluation, with a trend toward lower institutional rates for treatment subjects.

Burgener, Gilbert, and Mathy (2006) examined the effects of a multimodal intervention on people with early-stage Alzheimer's. With the brain plasticity theory as a basis for the intervention, an experimental design was used. Participants were randomly assigned to treatment ($N = 24$) or control ($N = 19$) groups, with a baseline mean Mini–Mental State Examination score of 22.5 across groups. The 20-week treatment group consisted of cognitive exercises, physical exercises, and a support group. Positive outcomes were found in all areas, including higher cognitive scores in the treatment group, improvement in physical balance, and evidence of improved self-esteem at the 20-week mark.

The TTAP Method is a multimodal approach founded on the psychological work of Arnold Lazarus (1989), developed in the 1950s and expanded using the concept of cognitive behavioral therapy. Lazarus was the first to introduce the term *behavior therapy* into the professional literature. Multimodal approaches grew out of the belief that effective treatment outcomes required moving away from more narrowly focused cognitive and behavioral methods and toward including physical sensations as distinct from emotional states (steps 1, 2, 3, 4, 5, 6, 8, and 9 of the TTAP Method); visual images (steps 2, 3, 4, 5, 6, 7, 8, and 9), which are distinct from language-based thinking; and the need for interpersonal relationships (each step of the TTAP Method).

The TTAP Method is based in art therapy and art recreation activities. The creative arts interactions are highly adaptable to the Alzheimer's population. The first two steps are the most significant in helping participants self-identify their needs through conversation, music, and meditation. (Chapter 3 discusses in more detail how to create interactions specifically for people with Alzheimer's.) The TTAP Method assists caregivers, therapists, and activity professionals in developing person-centered programming that effortlessly moves participants through a variety of creative arts activities and offers the following benefits:

- Allows for assessments, focusing on what is best for the person at any given moment and how his or her needs can be met at any stage of Alzheimer's

- Boosts self-esteem and enhances overall sense of self in the community

- Helps the person with dementia to continue to participate meaningfully in life

- Holistically supports one's functional capacity and life management in different phases of Alzheimer's disease

- Serves participants in a person-centered way and is timely and goal oriented

- Provides a mechanism for the discovery of the self through the creative process

- Increases social participation and integration of the individual into one-to-one interactions or group experiences

- Provides detailed protocols and documentation charts to demonstrate and track daily, weekly, and yearly therapeutic interactions

CONCLUSION

Expressive art therapies are a powerful healing tool. When used in traditional forms of functional intervention, they can help people release the stress that produces emotions that are known to cause immune system deficiency (Zatz & Goldstein, 1985). Expressive art can help people maintain and maximize the body's and the mind's ability to work harmoniously with any form of prescribed treatment. It can also help in the release of any negative thoughts and fears that can block the body's ability to heal physically, emotionally, and spiritually.

Clinics, adult day program centers, hospitals, rehabilitation facilities, long-term care facilities, and hospices in the United States and around the world are increasingly incorporating creative arts into the practice of patient care. A 2009 report titled State of the Field Report: Arts in Healthcare summarizes the results of two national surveys (State of the Field Committee, 2009). The findings indicate that half of health care institutions in the United States have arts programming and that the reported benefits include shorter hospital stays, reduced need for medications, and improved workplace satisfaction and employee retention. The most sophisticated universities and medical centers are now creating art–hospital programs that invite community artists to work with patients. The most significant factor is that it is not the product but the process that matters. Art, music, drama, poetry, and all other expressive therapies, when allowed to permeate the sterile and institutional environment in which the client lives, can open clients' hearts, minds, and spirits to the joys of self-expression and creativity.

TTAP Method Programming for People with Alzheimer's Disease

ccording to the U.S. Department of Labor's *Occupational Out-look Handbook, 2010–2011*, rapid growth in the number of older adults will spur job growth for art and recreation therapy professionals and paraprofessionals in assisted living facilities, adult day programs, and other social assistance agencies. Employment of art and recreation therapists or therapeutic recreation specialists is expected to increase 15% from 2008 to 2018, faster than the average for all other health field occupations. In nursing care facilities—the largest industry employing recreation therapists—employment will grow faster than the occupation as a whole as the number of older adults continues to grow (http://stats.bls.gov/oco/ocos082.htm).

Coupled with the rapid and steady growth in the number of older adults over the coming decades will be an escalation in the numbers of people diagnosed with Alzheimer's disease and other forms of dementia. As already noted, without a cure in sight, 16 million Americans are expected to have Alzheimer's by 2050, out of a projected 80 million people with the diagnosis worldwide (www.alz.org).

Job growth in the near future for art and recreation therapists will stem from the growing therapy needs of our aging population. The art and therapeutic recreation specialist faces the challenge of developing programming to meet the needs of this very special group of clients. One out of every three certified recreation therapists will work with older adults, according to the 2010 census taken by the American Therapeutic Recreation Association, and many of their clients will have cognitive and memory impairment. Unfortunately, many classes and formal training programs do not provide real hands-on directives for working with this group of individuals.

The TTAP Method® was first developed to engage older adults as a way to preserve cognitive functioning. This innovative, integrative approach to therapeutic recreation and creative arts programming has also proven effective in enhancing cognition and socialization for those with Alzheimer's (see Chapters 2, 5, and 7). In the late 1980s through the 1990s there was a complete void as to what type of therapeutic programs could be implemented successfully with this group. Common questions that art and recreation therapists, psychotherapists, and social workers ask regarding individuals with Alzheimer's disease include the following: Is there programming that can be done? Is the client able to remember enough to participate in an arts program? What if the client never participated in the creative arts? Could he or she now learn? All of these questions can be answered with one word: *Yes!* As discussed in Chapters 4 and 5, the brain can retain new information and create new ideas throughout the life span in response to learning, experiences, and the environment, including for those with Alzheimer's. The more stimulation the brain receives, the better it functions, even in the face of Alzheimer's. The essence of the TTAP Method programming for people with Alzheimer's lies in assessing the person's strengths and the weaknesses at whichever stage of the disease. The therapist then plans and adapts the interventions by incorporating the participants' abilities into the creative arts programming.

This chapter provides specific guidelines and approaches for therapists using the TTAP Method with individuals who have Alzheimer's, including suggestions for how to adapt programming for those in the mild, moderate, or severe stages of the disease process and variations for intergenerational programming.

DEFINITIONS IN ALZHEIMER'S

It is helpful for the therapist using the TTAP Method with people with Alzheimer's to understand some common problems associated with the disease.

Communication Disorder

Communication disorder, which is a condition of communication deterioration, starts from the onset of the disease. It interferes with a person's ability to understand the communication of others. Not understanding speech from others, especially in a group situation, can be very frustrating. It is helpful for the therapist to repeat or clarify the words or phrases of others to ensure that communication breakdown does not occur often.

Communication Breakdown

Communication breakdown occurs when the participant does not understand the words of the speaker at all (see Figure 1.4 in Chapter 1).

Multicultural groups are often found within therapeutic programs, which can be more difficult for participants with Alzheimer's because of varying dialects and pronunciations. The therapist must be sensitive to tones and word pronunciations to minimize the communication breakdown. Talking slowly and engaging the client through eye contact is important for successful communication. Communication breakdown can also be minimized by using graphic organizers. (See the discussion of descriptive patterning and graphic organizing tools in this chapter.) The therapist can refer to these tools often when discussing a topic or a theme.

Learned Helplessness

Learned helplessness, described by Seligman (1975), arises when an individual discovers through repeated experiences that his or her actions have little effect on the outcome of the situation, especially in the restricted environment of a nursing facility. Through the TTAP Method, the individual directly affects the group through participation and the act of doing and creating artwork. The active involvement of "doing" keeps the client continually feeling positive and valued, thus combating helplessness.

The actual TTAP Method programming sometimes has a very dramatic effect on family and staff, as individuals with Alzheimer's suddenly start to share very detailed information about their past, almost reliving moment by moment memories that have been buried by time. Through the TTAP Method individuals are continually asked to go within and remember, recall, and then share their vision through the mind's eye.

Window of Lucidity

A *window of lucidity* is a moment when an individual with Alzheimer's suddenly remembers something or talks more clearly about an idea that seemed to have been long forgotten. These can occur very unpredictably, but it is not unusual for windows of lucidity to occur when an individual is engaged in artistic or expressive activities. The TTAP Method offers two specific approaches for creating windows of lucidity: (1) through objects and sensory stimulation, and (2) through the use of body relaxation (meditation) and guided imagery. (See the discussion of meditation and guided imagery later in the chapter.) A therapist, for example, can hand a seashell to participants and then ask them to close their eyes and express what images come to mind (person, place, time), or what feelings the seashell gives them. In my experience it is incredible to hear the majority of participants express a profound emotional and meaningful memory. This simple but powerful activity of holding and feeling an object opens the subconscious to memories of people, places, and events that are deeply buried within the brains of people with Alzheimer's.

COMMUNICATION AS THE FIRST STEP IN THE TTAP METHOD

TTAP Method programming encourages rich language usage, which is crucial for maintaining self-esteem and quality of life for those with Alzheimer's. The first step of the TTAP Method is to conduct either a one-on-one or group conversation by introducing a theme or an object for the individual or group to focus on. For example, the therapist asks participants to reflect on and visualize past summer vacations and places that they have visited. From this simple directive, wonderful memories are brought to mind and the group members begin to name different cities and countries where they have experienced summer vacations. Participants share memories of warm summer days full of family, friends, and carefree experience. The therapist can then lead the group into a creative art activity. This simple yet powerful way in which to start communication has been proven time and time again to be very successful in engaging and focusing a group.

Communication has been identified as an important aspect of social support. Pizzaro (2004) found that during the process of making art, the artwork itself provides a medium of expression, communication, and mental stimulation that may ultimately assist in regenerating brain cells. The art process, which is nonverbal, can be a significant and positive stimulus for tapping into higher verbal regulatory functions that may be blocked or out of reach due to emotional stressors or disease processes, such as dementia (Snowdon, Kemper, Mortimer, Greiner, Wekstein & Markesbery, 1996; Bayle, Tomoeda & Trosset, 1992). Through increased social support systems some individuals will not progress to dementia and have the potential to improve or revert back to normal memory with early interventions (Golomb, Kluger, de Leon, Ferris, Mittelman, Cohen & George, 1996).

Alzheimer's and other forms of dementia cause a person's communication skills to deteriorate along a somewhat predictable course. This is often one of the largest challenges for the therapist. Deterioration of memory, understanding, speech, language, and social skills takes a toll on a client's ability to communicate effectively. Any therapist who has worked with individuals with Alzheimer's will agree that some days are better than others, and this is often confusing and frustrating for the therapist. The TTAP Method teaches art and recreation therapists to think differently about how to communicate with someone diagnosed with Alzheimer's. With each programming step the therapist constantly reaches out to each participant by asking open-ended questions geared toward the person's past (e.g., What did you do when you were a teenager on a hot summer day?).

In the early stage of Alzheimer's, a person starts to experience difficulty with describing short-term events. A therapist can develop a productive program by choosing a theme from the participants' past, such as weddings, and have them share something about a wedding in which they participated or about their own wedding. The ability to retrieve long-term memories, such as one's wedding day, is a strength that can be built on in thematic programming. Diamond (1999) confirmed that the ability to recall a positive experience activates the endorphins within the brain, thereby providing positive feelings, regenerating brain cells, and promoting a better quality of life.

The ability to structure a sentence properly remains intact even until late in the disease process (Santo Pietro & Ostuni 1997). Conversely, some skills, such as word finding, weaken almost from the beginning of the disease. With the right kind of support, however, the therapist can help the individual find the correct words to describe events. People diagnosed with Alzheimer's naturally strive, even in the face of the disease, to communicate and express themselves to those around them.

Communication breakdown is common in meeting the needs of people with Alzheimer's (Santo Pietro & Ostuni, 1997). Individuals with Alzheimer's struggle with the following seven issues, and being sensitive to these concerns enables better participation, less frustration, and more successful communication:

- Loss of independence

- Loss of social roles

- Loss of physical attractiveness and grooming skills

- Loss of energy

- Loss of family and friends

- Loss of familiar environments

- Loss of first-language partners

Similarly important to reiterate is that certain strengths and abilities are preserved throughout the disease progression and are incorporated into the TTAP Method (see Chapter 2, CCDERS Approach™), including the ability to

- Communicate with others

- Connect with others

- Differentiate likes and dislikes

- Express feelings and emotions

- Recall long-term memories

- Self-express (pleasurable emotions and receiving joy)

Caregivers and therapists can better understand and address the communication behaviors of individuals with Alzheimer's by realizing not what is lost during the disease process but, more important, what is preserved. Success in any therapeutic programming lies in using the abilities that the individual still has and ensuring that frustration, stress, and feelings of incompetence do not arise.

DESCRIPTIVE PATTERNING

In leading programs using the TTAP Method, the therapist begins to work with the participants to explore a theme first through conversation and then through creative brainstorming that is directed at a particular creative art experience with one central theme. The therapist accomplishes this by using an organizational system. Most declarative information that the group participants share can be organized using one of six standard patterns and their graphic representations: descriptive, process/causation, generalization, sequence, problem solving, and concept. These graphic organizing tools have been used throughout the United States in elementary and public school systems for organizing information in teaching since the mid-1990s. (See the discussion of graphic organizing tools in the next section.)

Descriptive patterning is a formalized way of displaying creative thinking with structured formats of charting. The charts can be enlarged on a blackboard or dry-erase board, and photocopies can be distributed to the participants (see Appendix D). The participants can follow along while the therapist documents the group's input in a large and easy-to-read format. Remember that writing, thinking, speaking, and doing all stimulate the brain.

The following is a detailed description of each type of organizational pattern:

1. *Descriptive patterns:* Descriptive patterns (see Figure 3.1A) can be used to organize facts or characteristics about specific people, places, things, and events. This is the simplest form of graphic display. The therapist gives each participant a copy to start working on a particular theme. If the chosen theme is holidays, for example, the therapist can ask each person to write down the four most significant holidays he or she can

remember. Then the therapist can display on the group chart the four most common holidays among the group and then direct the group in choosing one holiday to use as the theme.

2. *Process and causation patterns:* Process and causation patterns (see Figure 3.1B) can be used to organize information into a causal network that leads to a specific outcome or into a sequence of steps that lead to a specific product, idea, or elements of a theme. If the group has chosen making flowers as a theme for an art activity, then a process/causation chart can be used to organize the many different ways in which a flower can be made. For example, a flower can be made individually, then organized into a bunch, and then placed into an arrangement. This process is crucial when working with individuals with Alzheimer's as a way for the therapist to visually organize the participants' thoughts and thereby prevent frustration and anxiety.

3. *Generalization patterns:* Generalization patterns (see Figure 3.1C) organize information into generalized supporting information. This is a good diagram to use to back up theme information. This graphic organizer could be used to give examples of various cars that the clients owned or of types of trees that grow in various states.

4. *Sequence patterns:* Sequence patterns (see Figure 3.1D) organize events in a specific chronological order. If you were discussing events in history chronologically, then this would be an excellent graphic organizer. This is also an excellent cognitive tool to stimulate recall abilities.

5. *Problem-solving patterns:* Problem-solving patterns (see Figure 3.1E) organize information into an identified problem and its possible solutions. This is another excellent format for dealing with conflict or problems in that it gives the therapist direction in the narrative, and it gives the participants the ability to interact and be heard. A good example of problem solving is when two people who live together cannot adjust to the living environment. This technique can enable clients to work out living arrangements by identifying what is personally important to each one individually.

6. *Concept patterns:* Concept patterns (see Figure 3.1F) are the most general of all patterns. Like descriptive patterns, they deal with people, places, things, and events, but they represent an entire class or category and usually illustrate specific

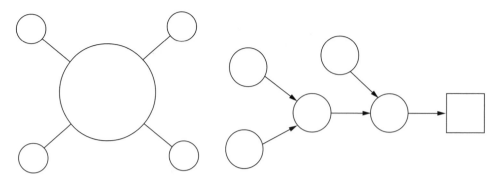

A. Descriptive patterns

B. Process and causation patterns

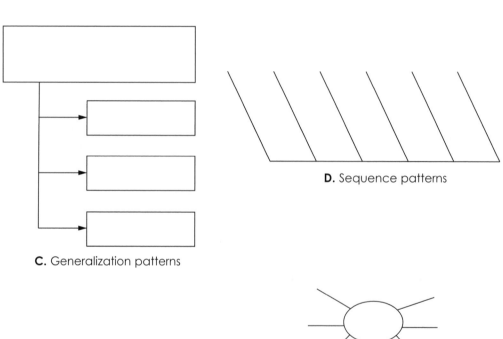

C. Generalization patterns

D. Sequence patterns

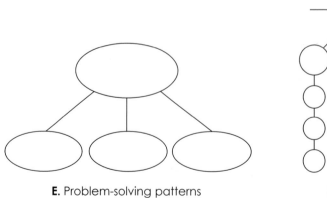

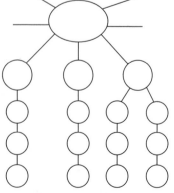

E. Problem-solving patterns

F. Concept patterns

Figure 3.1 (A–F).   Graphic organizing tools.

examples and defining characteristics of the concept. An example of using a concept pattern is to define a special evening event and all of the various foods needed.

Through the TTAP Method, this visual process creates a flow effect, or optimal experience, while also providing structure for the participants and allowing the therapist to expand the programs; the typical 45-minute session can be increased to an hour and a half. Each participant works on a personal experience while supporting the group. Increased verbalization occurs naturally because the person is being asked to share thoughts that are introspective and relevant and that hold significant meaning. This flow effect, or optimal experience, will occur during each phase of the programming (see Chapter 2).

GRAPHIC ORGANIZING TOOLS

There are many benefits to using graphic organizers as part of the group process. Graphic organizers can be as simple as a timeline or as complex as using clusters to formulate different ideas. The following is a breakdown of six reasons for and benefits of using graphic organizers to start a program:

1. The therapist can use a graphic organizer to illustrate and explain relationships between different topics that are discussed. The illustration and visual stimulation are enhanced by using an enlarged board to depict and define this material. The writing of the information can be designated to one of the group members, if possible, thereby stimulating the writing of words, phrases, and so forth.

2. The use of the organizer can depict information as a rewriting tool for effective lecture or information as well as demonstrations. For example, when leading a creative arts group writing session, the therapist can use the graphic organizer to focus and reflect on the theme for effective coverage of information. The therapist can also use it as a visual aid to reference. This is helpful when dealing with a topic that contains multiple components, such as how to work with clay or how to make enamel jewelry. This is ideal for clients with Alzheimer's.

3. Graphic organizers are used as a visual aid for participants who have cognitive problems, thereby ensuring visual learning while perceiving abstract ideas.

4. The therapist can use graphic organizers to assist clients who have a limited vocabulary. The number of people who have

immigrated to the United States has added a multicultural aspect to much of group programming. It is not rare to be in front of a group of clients who do not speak English as a first language or who do not speak English at all.

5. Graphic organizers can provide a visual representation of programs that will be linked through the theme. For example, the therapist might list which creative arts programs will be incorporated into the theme of traveling around the world.

6. Graphic organizers can be used to design monthly programs, bulletin boards, announcements, and various media presentations to the group, facility, or center. If the theme of spring were being used, for example, then a calendar could be designed in programming that holds meaning for the participants.

The clients derive a direct benefit from using a graphic organizer. It enhances visual and verbal skills that often diminish as an individual ages as well as stimulates the brain and thereby cell growth through the sharing and writing down of words and thoughts. A significant role of the graphic organizer is to organize ideas that the group is expressing and sharing; a graphic chart is used to keep a record of shared thoughts of all of the participants. When using a graphic organizer with a group, it is beneficial for all participants to share at least one idea, thereby increasing participation while enhancing self-esteem through the therapeutic experience.

The following describes the benefits that clients derive from using graphic organizers:

1. Clients can record on their own graphic chart relationships that are being shared in the program. Just as the therapist benefits from the writing, so can the clients.

2. Clients can use a graphic organizer to organize abstract thoughts before sharing or participating in a discussion. Clients can list and organize thoughts and ideas for their inquiry.

3. Graphic organizers can be used as a pre-discussion information tool. Clients can record thoughts or ideas that come to mind during a meditative session or while listening to music.

4. Graphic organizers can help clients manage their own thought process while recording how and what comes to mind first.

5. Graphic organizers can help clients prepare suggestions that they might have for presentations or display boards.

6. The most significant elements for clients are to enhance memory and writing skills, stimulate visual and auditory recognition, and support cognitive functioning and brain wellness.

STIMULATING PROCEDURAL MEMORIES THROUGH THE TTAP METHOD

The individual with Alzheimer's begins to lose memory for words, information, and events, but *procedural memory*, which is the knowledge of how to perform tasks, remains relatively intact until the late stages of dementia. Anderson (1990) explained that procedural memory is like a computer program; other types of memories are like separate forms of memory data stored within the computer. Individuals with moderate Alzheimer's do not know where they are going, but they remember how to walk. They do not wash their own clothes anymore, but give them fabric, soap, and water and they will wash. Similarly, they might not know what they are saying, but they can still speak. Other examples of procedural memories include folding clothes, pouring a glass of water, setting the table, washing hands, and passing plates.

The TTAP Method incorporates procedural memories into thematic programming. For example, a therapist can develop an activity using the themes *objects* or *seasons* to tap into a participant's procedural memory by assisting the individual to connect a memory through an object or season. Using food as a theme is another great method for eliciting procedural memories from individuals with Alzheimer's. Food is one of the most essential elements of life, starting from birth and ending at death. The following are examples of how the therapist can integrate the theme of food into programming:

- Discuss which types of food are eaten for various meals. Plan a meal with the participants. This can include designing a menu, choosing the foods, and, most significant, preparing food. The use of plastic utensils is important. Cutting foods such as bananas, melons, and breads is easy, and the participant derives much pleasure from the successful event.

- Counting is another interesting and creative way to use food. String beans; peanuts; jelly beans; and apples, pears, and any other fruit with seeds can be distributed among the participants, and then participants can be instructed to count objects or the seeds. Make this a challenge game, and give prizes for the winner. Next, have participants cut up the food for a salad or to cook.

- Food for Thought is a simple activity that asks the group to think about various foods and then add personal stories that are related to the foods. Cultural foods such as Chinese dim sum, Jewish pastries, Cuban rice and beans, and Italian ices or fresh mozzarella and tomatoes can be used for this type of procedural activity. In this creative program food is used as the creative object as well as a tasty treat! Food for Thought is a great way to motivate participation and enhance social interactions. (Food for Thought programming came out of the work of Janet Larghi, M.S., CTRS, the author [Linda Levine Madori, Ph.D.], and the Cabrini Nursing Home in New York City.)

Using the theme *facts* can also stimulate procedural memories in many different ways, including the following:

- Using the visualization board, ask participants to list facts about a common item, such as clothes. Have participants list various components of clothing, such as buttons, zippers, clasps, and so forth, then bring in samples of these components and have participants operate the items.

- The theme of facts can also be specific to performing tasks. Have participants visualize how they dance or exercise. Then have them act out the movements of these familiar acts. Revisiting old memories in this way can contribute significantly to the overall well-being of the participants.

Overall, the important goals to keep in mind when developing thematic programming for people with Alzheimer's disease include the following:

- Enhance participants' quality of life.

- Develop activities that participants can still do.

- Foster in participants a feeling of control over their environment.

- Enhance participants' self-esteem through therapeutic art and recreation experiences.

- Provide multiple opportunities for participant self-expression.

THE TTAP METHOD FOR PEOPLE WITH ALZHEIMER'S DISEASE

The following are general descriptions of the steps of the TTAP Method for people with Alzheimer's and other dementias:

Step 1: From individual thought to group conversation. Emphasis is on individual experiences from the past: vacations, holidays, family, religion, culture, traditions, life lessons, fashion, movies, and life problems and solutions. A word board or chart is an excellent visual tool for individuals with Alzheimer's, who may experience difficulties processing language in spoken form.

Step 2: From group conversation to music and meditation. Emphasis is on music of the specific time period or music of personal preferences that were derived from and support the theme of step 1. This population flourishes with musical stimulation. Play a piece of music from a favorite movie or Broadway show.

Step 3: From music and meditation to drawing and painting. Emphasis is on building on the image that emerges from the music. Use the active and responsive social abilities that these individuals still have. If multiple images emerge, then use them in collages, diagrams, and landscapes.

Step 4: From drawing and painting to sculpture. Emphasis is on projecting the theme into any form of abstract art made with clay, wire, or paper. There are no "mistakes"; everything created is of value.

Step 5: From sculpture to movement and dance. Emphasis is on connecting the theme to objects that can be used in a movement or dance program. Images can also be used for participants to act out or express a theme through movement.

Step 6: From movement and dance to group writing experience (poetry, stories). Emphasis is on connecting words, feelings, and phrases through writing (rhyming, storytelling).

Step 7: From group writing experience to food experience. Emphasis is on connecting the words, feelings, and phrases to foods that fit the theme subject(s).

Step 8: From food experience to theme event. Emphasis is on connecting all of the themes that were derived throughout the program and using, for example, the paintings to decorate the walls, the sculptures for centerpieces, and the food to make a meal for the participants.

Step 9: From theme event to phototherapy. Emphasis is on using photographs to stimulate memories and to capture each individual in a photograph for use in a future creative arts activity (collages, a group writing experience).

Step 10: From phototherapy to sensory stimulation. Emphasis is on connecting the senses to the theme.

Step 11: From sensory stimulation to drama or theater experience. Emphasis is on connecting the theme to a dramatic theater story or performance.

Step 12. Client feedback, assessment, and evaluation. Emphasis is on gathering client feedback through verbal questionnaires, which is crucial in assessing the satisfaction of the participants and the success of the TTAP Method programming in stimulating brain functioning and enhancing physical, spiritual, cognitive, emotional, and social capacity.

A significant goal of the TTAP Method is to provide the participant with all types of creative arts experiences. These goals are accomplished by using connected, creative activities around a theme to provide a stimulating and rich group experience for the participants. The order in which the steps are discussed in this chapter does not need to be followed in practice; the order can be changed or steps can be repeated to best suit each participant's needs and desires.

The sections that follow offer programming adaptation for people with mild, moderate, or severe Alzheimer's for each step of the TTAP Method. Each program begins with the therapist guiding the group in conversation about the activity theme (step 1). The therapist next leads the group through a music and meditation exercise (step 2), to relax the participants as well as focus them on the activity theme. The group is then led through a creative art activity (sculpture, group writing experience, theme event, etc.). Each TTAP Method program ends with the therapist gathering client feedback, assessment, and evaluation (step 12).

STEP 1. CONVERSATION

TTAP Method programming begins with conversation around a theme. For example, a good theme to use for those diagnosed with mild Alzheimer's is the current season. Once a theme has been chosen, the therapist then chooses a graphical organizational tool to focus the participants on the theme and to develop the theme into different types of creative arts activities. After gathering thoughts and ideas from participants about the theme, the therapist can then move on to the music and meditation (guided imagery) activity (step 2). For those participants diagnosed with early-stage Alzheimer's, therapists are advised to begin by focusing the conversation on describing what the TTAP Method is and then asking the participants if they have ever experienced a meditation or guided imagery. Those with mild Alzheimer's will also appreciate the therapist sharing with them that the creative arts experiences they are about to participate in have been proven to stimulate the brain and cognitive functioning.

STEP 2. MUSIC AND MEDITATION

After all participants have shared in conversation their thoughts about a chosen theme, the therapist next introduces a music and meditation exercise to relax and focus the participants. To begin to use music in thematic programming, introduce sounds, singing, records, tapes, and CDs that offer a connection to the theme. Using the theme of seasons, the therapist might introduce the sounds of the ocean for developing a summer theme. Once a piece of music has been selected, the therapist can lead the participants through a guided imagery exercise, using the music as a backdrop (Box 3.1). If you initially do not feel comfortable reading from the script, practice on friends and family before guiding your clients through the exercise.

For individuals with mild Alzheimer's, ask them to get comfortable in their chair and tell them that you are going to take them on a journey into their own special garden. After the meditation has been completed, discuss and share what each participant experienced. What memories were evoked; what thoughts or feelings came to mind? The next step is to use what the individuals saw, felt, or remembered in the next creative art experience.

This one experience uses the sensory cortex (feeling) to remember the feelings of the meditation. The occipital lobe (seeing) is stimulated by internal visualization of the guided imagery. The reticular formation (arousal) is stimulated by the thought process and positive stimulation of endorphins in the mind and the body. The temporal lobe (hearing) is stimulated by the music as well as the voice of the therapist. While the clients share their individual insights, Broca's area (speech) is being stimulated.

For individuals with severe or late-stage Alzheimer's, the guided imagery can be used successfully. You do not need to read the entire meditation script. Instead you can have the individual close his or her eyes and just visualize what the garden would be like. Ask questions such as Did you ever have a special garden? What would you do in your garden? What flowers, trees, and bushes grow in your garden? You might also want to bring in pictures of different gardens mounted on construction paper to try and elicit feedback about the images. Any information shared or remembered can be used as "windows" into further communication.

Box 3.1.   Exercise using guided imagery and music.

Close your eyes and take three deep breaths. With each inhaled breath, imagine calm and cleansing air flowing into your lungs. With each inhale, visualize releasing all negative feelings and stressors from your body; imagine clean and calming air flowing into your lungs. Feel your chest and diaphragm moving up and down.

Pause.

Count to five.

1. You are becoming more aware of your body relaxing.

2. Your eyes are starting to feel heavy.

3. You are feeling more relaxed than ever.

4. You see a garden door before you.

5. Open the door and walk through the gate *(garden door can be made of anything)*

Listen to the sounds being heard. What images come to mind? What people do you see? What kind of feelings do you have?

Pause.

Now, imagine that this garden has a beautiful forest full of old trees. You are walking in the forest, feeling completely at peace with yourself. You are exactly where you should be, right here, right now.

Pause.

I want you to imagine in your mind's eye a beautiful spot in this garden. Visualize sitting down, becoming very comfortable. Now, for the next 5 minutes *(or longer, depending on the group's abilities)*, relax and let your mind go. Let your thoughts come and go. If you feel as though you are falling asleep, it's okay. Just relax.

Pause for allotted time, no speaking.

Now, visualize yourself getting up. Walk back through the woods. Come up on the path. Now, walk toward the garden door, take one last look at this beautiful place, your special place, to which you can always come back in the morning before you arise or at night before you go to sleep.

Count backward.

5. You are starting to feel yourself.

4. You are becoming more aware of your body.

3. You are starting to feel and move your fingers.

2. Your eyes are feeling lighter.

1. Stretch and open your eyes.

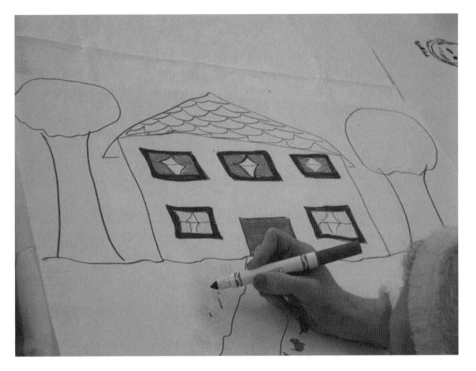

Figure 3.2. A resident draws her family home.

STEP 3. DRAWING AND PAINTING

After participating in the music and meditation (guided imagery) session, the clients have very clear images in their mind's eye. The therapist can give participants colored pencils, watercolors, markers, and tempera paints to move the images from the mind's eye to paper by asking the clients to draw or paint what they remember from the meditation. If the group is scheduled only once a day or once a week, the therapist can refresh clients' memories by playing the music that was used in the guided imagery in the background during the drawing and painting activity. There are many ways in which to conduct this process to stimulate memories for those with mild or moderate Alzheimer's. Most individuals are very intimidated by the pencil, so the therapist may want to start by using magazines that the clients can pick images from to cut out and glue onto paper. The therapist can ask participants to draw around the photograph so that the empty page is not an intimidation factor in the creative process.

For those with moderate Alzheimer's, the therapist can assist participants in moving images in the mind's eye to the page by asking them to pick colors they remember from the meditation versus asking them to draw an image. Another variation with this population is to place images cut from a magazine on the table along with glue sticks. Ask the participants to pick the images that most clearly identify the theme of what they saw in their garden. Yet another variation is supplying participants with colored shapes of tissue paper and asking them to choose the colors that best represent their garden, then assisting with gluing the shapes to the page.

If the conversation from the guided imagery exercise moves into a group theme, where, for example, the participants end up speaking about how they have all traveled to Italy at some point in their lives, the therapist can use this theme to engage the group in a drawing or painting activity. Have the participants create a group two-dimensional large canvas of Italy, or provide them with photographs from which to choose the ones that best fit their experiences in and memories of Italy. The TTAP Method is unique in that the group can decide where the next activity should be directed to meet their personal interests, or the therapist can facilitate ideas that have been expressed by the group. This is the fundamental strength of the approach—the group, the individual, and the therapist have a fundamental balance and function.

For someone with severe Alzheimer's, the therapist can move from trying to engage the person to share his or her thoughts about gardens via the guided imagery exercise to encouraging the person to share what might be in his or her personal garden. This can be done by showing the individual different images of flowers, chairs, water fountains, and trees. Have the person pick what tree, flower, or water fountain is in his or her special garden. To complete this activity, the therapist can assist the individual in gluing the chosen images to a large piece of colored construction paper. The therapist can then hang the piece of art in the client's room for the person to see.

In the process of going from imagination to image, the frontal lobe (problem solving) is one of the active components at work. The motor cortex (moving) is needed for the fine and gross motor skills of cutting, pasting, and drawing. The parietal lobe (touching) is stimulated by the manipulation of art materials, such as feeling the paper and other materials. The occipital lobe (seeing) is stimulated by the activity in the environment. The reticular formation (arousal) is stimulated by the identification with the process of making art and self-esteem. Individuals feel good about themselves when they are participating in an activity that is meaningful. Broca's area (speech) is active as a result of the social element in the creative arts group process. Imagery is the body's and the mind's inner language; art is the voice and expression of that nonverbal language. Using art can enable the individual to connect, possibly for the first time, to an emotion or an event that has not been thought of for decades. It can also stimulate emotional healing through the connection of deep and innermost feelings.

Processing Artwork with Your Clients

The therapist's responsibility in stimulating and motivating the group to verbalize about their artwork is to be a facilitator, coach, or guide, not an interpreter, as well as to be present emotionally and physically. Most successful group experiences occur when the therapist has provided a safe environment in which the participants feel comfortable to share their thoughts and inner feelings with the group and with the therapist.

Once the group has completed a creative arts activity, encourage participants to share with the group what they have created. Sharing feelings, experiences, memories, and creations is an integral component of the group process using the TTAP Method. Some people will be more willing to share than others. One way to encourage sharing is to change the physical seating arrangement. If clients are at individual desks, then rearrange the chairs in a circle. The circle represents the group, and every member of the group makes up and completes the circle.

Always allow clients to opt out of sharing their work if they choose. Respecting the individual's needs is extremely important to the process of making art, expressing oneself, and fostering self-esteem. Remember that each individual is taking something deep within him- or herself and putting it "out there" for everyone to see. This can be extremely difficult for some people, yet with continual positive feedback from the therapist, trust develops between the individual and the therapist as well as between the individual and the group.

The therapist focuses conversation on the common elements and continually encourages conversation within the group. The therapist's role is to listen and to synthesize creatively the images and information shared by the participants to reach the next level. Asking questions of the group is effective. Open-ended questions that do not elicit a yes or no response are ideal to encourage conversation. As the therapist looks around at everyone's work, he or she should take notice of what they have in common. Are there common colors that have been used by everyone? What are common elements among the artwork (e.g., are airplanes in every picture)? The therapist can use these commonalities to move to another theme within the group. The themes that emerge will also help the therapist to choose a next step in the TTAP Method to engage the group (drawing and painting, sculpture, movement and dance, group writing, food experience, or theme event).

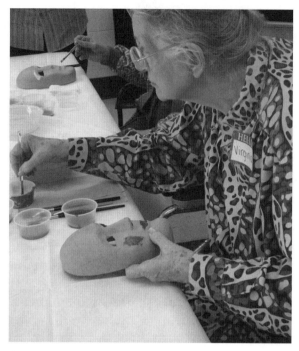

Figure 3.3. A resident uses watercolors as part of a mask-making program.

Expressing emotions through color, form, shape, and image releases memories that can be positive, but they can also be negative. Be prepared to handle feelings of loss or sorrow that might be expressed. If an individual in the group does experience a sorrowful memory, the therapist can take steps to promote feelings of safety and comfort. First, ask the individual whether he or she would like to share the memory. If the person wants to talk with the group, then promote the sharing. If he or she does not want to talk, then make sure that the person is not left alone. Have a nurse, family member, or staff member comfort the person in private. Often, people cry to express feelings of sorrow over a loved one.

Once all participants have completed their work, the therapist can mount for display each client's work, or the group can cut out parts of each person's finished work to create a group collage/mural. This technique works well when you have participants with varying abilities. Always finish any artwork with framing, matting, or mounting, and label clients' names in a professional manner. Remember, the way in which the therapist handles and displays artwork will be reflected in the way that others will view and respect the work. Also, participants feel a great sense of accomplishment and pride when communicating about their artwork with family members.

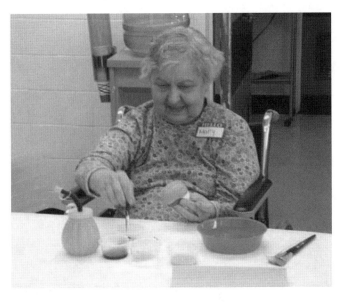

Figure 3.4. A resident participating in a sculpture program evidences fine motor coordination, cognitive concentration, and overall enjoyment.

STEP 4. SCULPTURE

For those with mild Alzheimer's, a sculpture activity can be done as an individual project within the group project. Participants can create a range of three-dimensional sculpture pieces using materials ranging from papier-mâché to clay to wire to sticks and even to objects found in the kitchen, such as paper plates, plastic straws, and plastic spoons. The garden theme can still be used, or the theme can move into a special garden a participant experienced growing up (a grandparents' farm, large fields of gardens, a childhood garden). Participants in a sculpture activity as part of a Cornell University study of the use of the TTAP Method with individuals with mild Alzheimer's created beautiful colored floral centerpieces that were inspired by their conversations about gardens, which led to a theme of favorite flowers through their lives. The group decided they wanted to create their own centerpieces by using artificial flowers placed into inexpensive clay flower pots. Another activity could be to bring in colored tissue paper and have participants make flowers and then create centerpieces or bouquets of flowers.

This activity can be adapted to individuals with moderate Alzheimer's by giving participants Sculpey™ (a self-hardening clay) or Play-Doh™ and asking them to sculpt a flower, water fountain, or special tree that they remember from a garden. Participants might ask the therapist for help in doing this activity, which is perfectly fine—we all

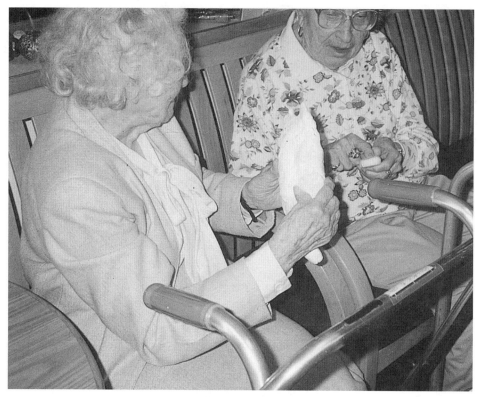

Figure 3.5. Social stimulation is essential for overall well-being. These two individuals share thoughts as part of a group sculpture program.

ask for and need help, and the arts is a place where assistance should always be given. Another variation is to use already-made tissue flowers and have the participants attach the flowers to the stems. Also have leaves ready so that each group member can pick how many leaves should be placed on a stem.

For individuals with severe Alzheimer's, you might want to bring in fresh flowers. (Be careful first to find out about any allergies from the nursing staff.) Have the person smell and touch the flowers. Ask questions such as: What does the smell remind you of? Where have you seen this flower before? Do you like this flower? What is your favorite flower? Assist the person in creating a centerpiece for the room. The therapist can also bring in paper flowers and ask the individual to choose which ones he or she likes and then assist the person in making a personal bouquet, wall hanging, or door decoration.

Creating sculptures engages the sensory cortex (feeling) through sensations from the sculpture itself as well as the materials used. The occipital lobe (seeing) is stimulated by the external visualization of the

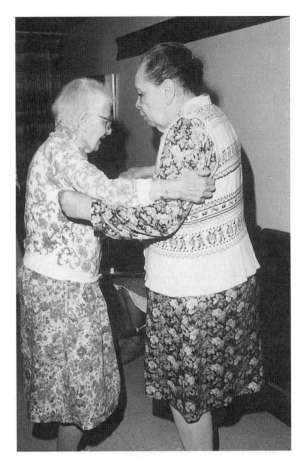

Figure 3.6. Two women enjoy a dance and movement program.

process. The thought processes and positive stimulations of endorphins in the mind and the body engage the reticular formation (arousal). The temporal lobe (hearing) is stimulated by the group's ongoing conversations as well as by the therapist's voice. And as the participants share their individual insights, Broca's area (speech) is stimulated.

STEP 5. MOVEMENT AND DANCE

With a movement and dance activity based on the chosen theme, the therapist introduces an object, or prop, by which to motivate the participants to move.

Movement and dance programming can provide individuals with mild or moderate Alzheimer's opportunities to be physically and socially active. Movement also enables each individual to express feelings and emotions in a relaxed and safe group environment. It is important to keep your clients moving and involved in physical activities.

Current research has shown the therapeutic benefits of physical activity on memory and cognitive functioning. In a study, for example, of the effects of exercise on people with mild Alzheimer's disease who were age 60 or older, those who were physically active had less atrophy in key areas of the brain associated with memory (Basler, 2008). The findings of the study suggest that cardiovascular activity may help slow the progress of the disease progression. One theory as to why is that cardiovascular activity maintains healthy blood flow to the brain as people age (McKeever 2009).

A growing movement program incorporates yoga, whether in a chair or in a wheelchair. Simple yoga stretches can be used to create a movement program. The deep breathing and gentle movement of yoga have been shown to enhance blood circulation and joint movement as well as decrease arthritic pain. The key is adaptation; make sure you adapt for each individual in the group.

Using Props in Movement Programs

Motivation is a continual challenge, and the use of props can motivate movement within the group experience. When beginning a movement program for individuals with mild or moderate Alzheimer's, the therapist should introduce an object, or prop, first and then ask the participants to move their bodies. This order is less threatening, and greater group cohesiveness can be achieved. The following props have been successful in beginning a movement group program:

Balls, Balloons, and Frisbees. Use balls, balloons, and Frisbees for warm-up exercising, alone or in conjunction with music. Objects take the individual's mind off of the body and project focus onto the object, thereby providing a feeling of security and safety. Objects are also a good way to have participants introduce themselves; they state their name while holding the object, then throw it to the next person in the group. Using the object in competition is another good warm-up; pass the object to the beat of the music, and see how long it can be tossed before falling.

Scarves. The use of scarves can stimulate and motivate the most difficult groups. The movement of fabric is a good point of departure to moving into body movements. Long pieces of fabric can be bought from a fabric store as remnants and are not costly. These colorful pieces of fabric lower the participants' resistance so that they can be directed to move different parts of the body. Fabrics also work well when orchestrating the group to move together as a whole to form a cohesive group experience.

Musical Instruments. The therapist can use musical instruments to introduce music that has different beats. Instrumental use is also a good way to find each person's personality within the group. This can be achieved by having each member play his or her own rhythm or beat and having the other members of the group repeat and prolong the beat. Another directive is to have individuals add their own ending to the last person's beat, thereby creating an entirely new musical rhythm.

Audiotapes, CDs, and Portable Music Devices. Music can be easily incorporated into movement and dance programming. Nature sounds, African drumming, and the rhythms of Brazilian music, for example, can be used creatively to enhance the group experience, motivate participants, and encourage discussion.

Common Exercise Equipment. Many different exercise products can be used in music and movement programming. Weighted balls, elastic bands, and weight belts for feet and arms can all be used in the group experience.

Movement, and Now Dance!

The therapist can start a movement and dance session with a discussion of what took place during the previous session. Remember that continual conversation and interaction enhance cognitive functioning. The primary goal of the movement and dance component of programming is to motivate movement by fostering self-expression. This self-expression, represented in dance format, can be very exciting for older adults because dance was one of the only "real" recreational activities that was free and socially accepted during the first part of the 20th century. When incorporating music into programming it is essential that the therapist research what the members of the group enjoy listening to, which composers they listened to as young adults, who their favorite singers were, which musicians or singers they had the chance to see in concert. You will be surprised at the answers you might uncover, and the participants will feel more motivated to move hearing familiar sounds and voices from the past.

Continuing with a garden theme, the therapist can find pieces of music with sounds of nature, wind, water, or the like to develop a movement and dance program for individuals with mild Alzheimer's. Have the participants sit in a circle, hand each a colorful scarf, long piece of cloth, or streamer, and have them wave the object at different times to the rhythm of the music playing in the background.

For individuals with moderate Alzheimer's, again using music in the background, ask the participants to move as the sound; be the wind, be a seagull, fly in the sky. Another good adaptation is to show the group a dance musical via DVD and have the participants move along to the music. Simple instruments such as drums are also very helpful in motivating individuals to move their hands, arms, and legs.

Movement and dance programming can also be adapted for people with severe Alzheimer's. The therapist, for example, can beat two drum sticks and encourage the person to move just his or her fingers or hands. Music can still resonate with this population. A client may have enjoyed listening and dancing to the music of Frank Sinatra as a younger adult. The therapist can play a Sinatra tune and encourage the person to tap his or her feet.

The use of objects or props in the experience of movement and dance stimulates the sensory cortex (touching). The occipital lobe (seeing) is stimulated by the external visualization of the process that the participants are witnessing and engaging in. The thought processes and release of endorphins in the mind and the body positively stimulate the reticular formation (arousal). The temporal lobe (hearing) is stimulated by the music, the group's conversations, and the voice of the therapist. Broca's area (speech) is stimulated as the participants share their individual likes, dislikes, thoughts, and feelings.

STEP 6. GROUP WRITING EXPERIENCE

Olders adults of the early 20th century are of a generation that used the written word to communicate. Words, poems, and storytelling grow naturally out of a music/meditation, sculpture, or drawing/painting program. Artwork that group members have created can be used to express feelings and life stories through the written word that the participants associate with the programming theme.

To begin a group writing experience (step 6), first revisit the theme by listening to music that was played as part of the guided imagery exercise or that was played in the background as part of a movement and dance session the group may already have participated in. Then ask the participants to come up with a list of words that they associate with the theme. The therapist can also revisit the theme with the group by reviewing the word board that was created as part of step 1 to focus the participants on the chosen theme. It is important to have notebooks, binders, or some other form of bound paper so that participants who are still able to write can keep whatever they write in

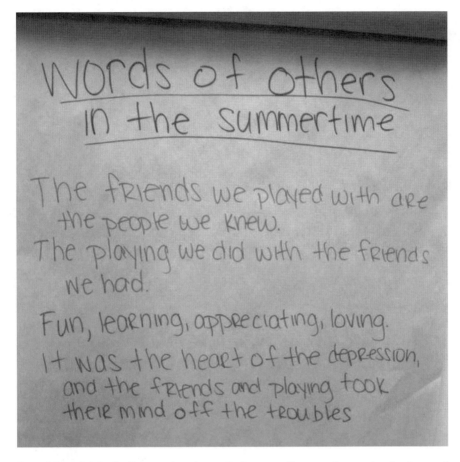

Figure 3.7.   A brief reflection composed as part of group writing experience using the theme of summertime.

the same place. After participants have created a free-flowing list of words, the therapist can ask them one-by-one to share their best three words with the group. Then, using the format of who, what, where, when, and how, the therapist can guide the group in using the words to create sentences and finally a poem or story that relates to the theme. A variation for people who have mild dementia is for each person to write one sentence and then have the group put the sentences together as one story or poem.

Creating the free-flowing list of words is an exercise that works well for individuals with mild or moderate Alzheimer's. The therapist may need to organize the words to some degree. For those with mild Alzheimer's, using artwork that the group created as part of previous session (photo collage, drawing/painting, sculpture), the therapist can ask the participants to describe what they see and write down words that can be used to create a title for their art pieces. Using the titles, the

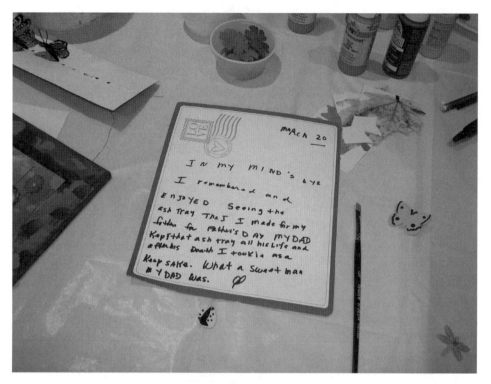

Figure 3.8. A personal reflection using the theme of Father's Day written on a large postcard following a guided imagery session.

therapist can then guide the group in creating a story about their pieces of art. The titled artworks with their written story can be displayed for each member of the group to see, reflect on, and be proud of.

Another activity for those with mild Alzheimer's is to ask the group to share in writing a story based on an event from their past that relates to the theme. Life stories hold enriching tales of wisdom. Sharing these stories can create bonds that will continue after the therapist leaves the program, and it allows all individuals to experience themselves but also to experience themselves in others. Recognizing common responses to life's ups and downs brings people closer together. These stories are a window into the past and offer the individual another moment to relive a great experience, for themselves and for the others.

For participants with moderate Alzheimer's, use a large white or black board or large paper chart to document the free-flowing list of words that the group can then use to write a poem or story. These individuals are better able to follow their thought processes when they can see the words that they have said as well as those that others have said. This process is an effective cognitive rehabilitation exercise that can be repeated after each step of the TTAP Method.

Those with severe Alzheimer's have often lost the ability to form words, while others can occasionally utter simple words or phrases. There are many stories, however, of a relative or caregiver of someone in the last stages of the disease who starts a conversation with the person, and he or she almost seems to "wake up" for a few minutes and actually utters coherent words in response. Science has so much still to discover about the brain and its functioning, so always try and then try again. And always bring an object of personal meaning for the person to see and touch (a favorite picture or vase from the person's home), and see if you can elicit a verbal or nonverbal response.

The group writing experience stimulates the sensory cortex (feeling), in the touch and feel of the writing materials. The external visualization of the poem or story being written stimulates the occipital lobe (seeing). The reticular formation (arousal) is stimulated by the thought processes and positive stimulation of endorphins in the mind and the body. The group's ongoing conversations and the voice of the therapist stimulate the temporal lobe (hearing). While the participants share their individual insights, Broca's area (speech) is being stimulated.

STEP 7. FOOD EXPERIENCE

People socialize around eating while connecting emotionally to family and friends throughout the life span. Food is a significant part of various cultures, religions, and holidays. An excellent theme for creative programming, food can be used for activities involving counting; creating; mixing; cutting; distinguishing textures; categorizing by animal, mineral, or vegetable; sorting by color or shape; and so forth. Food truly affects all senses (taste, touch, smell, sight, and hearing). A room full of strangers can be brought together by talking about food, touching and feeling different foods, preparing food, and using food in innovative ways in therapeutic programming. (With any food programming, the therapist must be very careful to ask staff and family members about all food restrictions or allergies.)

Continuing with the garden theme, if you are working with individuals who have mild Alzheimer's, have the group discuss what foods they would like to include in a garden picnic basket or picnic lunch. Organize getting the items, and if you are working with independent individuals you can go shopping with them for the items. The next activity would be to prepare part of or, if possible, the entire picnic menu. If the group wants to prepare sandwiches, shop for the components and then have the participants put them together.

Food events are celebratory and can be shared with family members as well as caregivers or staff. Ask the group to brainstorm what special food event they would like to create. A director of a community

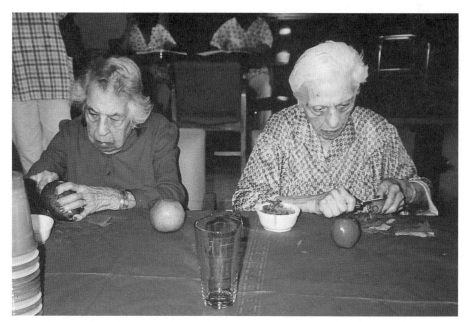

Figure 3.9. Residents cut and prepare apples for a pie.

day center shared with me that her group chose to create a Valentine's Day party in the summer. She arranged for the group to make cookies shaped and decorated as hearts and arrows. The participants were then asked to write a poem for someone they love, to decorate it, and to give it to that loved one (grandchild, wife, son). The director also played romantic music in the background and led the group in a dancing activity. Valentine's Day can be a day of love anytime, any month, anywhere.

Food events for those with moderate Alzheimer's can also be very exciting and rewarding. The sights, smells, and tastes of foods trigger many memories. Food programming can be adapted to strengthen cognitive functioning. The therapist, for example, can begin a food program using Food for Thought. The foods that the group chooses can be used for adding, subtracting, guessing who has the most, and so forth. Continuing with the garden theme, if the group chooses to include fruits with their picnic, the therapist can lead them in making a fruit salad. Hand a paper plate to each person as well as a bunch of grapes. Start by asking each participant to guess who has the most grapes in their bunch. Then ask the group to pull apart their grapes from the vine and count them. This activity is excellent for cognitive and social stimulation; not only are people talking to each other, but they are also guessing and counting, which engage different regions of the brain. Then ask the participants to place their grapes into a large bowl that will become the fruit salad for the lunch. Next, give each person a banana and ask the group what favorite recipes of theirs use bananas. Did they eat them in sandwiches, like Elvis Presley did? Were they included in their lunch boxes? Pass out plastic knives and have the participants cut up the bananas and then place them into the large bowl. This activity can be repeated using whichever fruits are available or in season (blueberries, strawberries, apples), continuing the conversation using the same cues and questions about each fruit.

Food can be a bit more difficult to use with individuals with severe Alzheimer's. One variation would be to approach the theme by using foods that have held meaning in the person's life. For example, if the family shares that their loved one always enjoyed red wine or port, bring in a bottle to stimulate these memories. If the person lived in an inner city and enjoyed foods from street venders, bring some roasted peanuts, popcorn, or candies for the person to touch, smell, or taste to stimulate memories and conversation. Another adaption is to transcribe the recipe for a dish that the person was famous for cooking. Ask the individual about the special pie she would make for Thanksgiving, which ingredients she used, and how she would prepare it. This activity can stimulate recall of procedural memories related to preparing the pie or any other recipes the individual might recall. Memories associated with the holiday or other food event might also be recalled (times spent eating with family and friends).

Food programming stimulates the sensory cortex (feeling) in the tastes, smells, and feel of the foods and ingredients. The occipital lobe (seeing) is stimulated by the external visualization of the process of preparing food. The thought processes and release of endorphins in the mind and the body positively stimulate the reticular formation (arousal). The temporal lobe (hearing) is stimulated by the group's conversations and the voice of the therapist. As the participants share their individual insights and memories of their favorite foods, Broca's area (speech) is stimulated.

STEP 8. THEME EVENT

Almost every facility, adult day center, hospital, or rehabilitation center holds parties and celebrations of special events. Using a theme event (holiday, cultural, birthday) is a great way to display all of the group's efforts throughout the programming. Centerpieces can come out of a sculpture program. Pictures for the walls can come out of a drawing and painting program. Table dressings, including creative napkin rings and placemats, can come out of a food program. A musical selection can come from a movement and dance program.

Ask the group what would be the best music for the theme event. Show a movie that depicts a special time of year that the event is high-

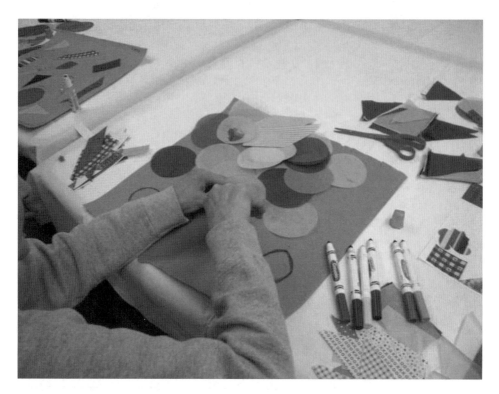

Figure 3.10.   A woman creates a collage of different shapes and colors using fabrics that the therapist will then help her frame and hang in her room.

lighting. Individuals can create murals on windows using watercolor paints to enhance the event.

A Food for Thought program can be used to organize the food and create the shopping list for the theme event. The group can create thematic invitations and menus for the guests. Some facilities, such as long-term care and assisted living, allow residents to prepare their own food.

Special events are another way to bring the community into the program. Invite family members and friends to the events to show them how the creative arts enhance the quality of life of the participants. Events are also a good time to encourage people who might be interested in joining the programming group to participate.

Theme events can easily be linked to the weather, a season, a holiday, or a cultural event. If you choose a weather or holiday theme, be sure it coincides with the actual season taking place for those you are working with who have moderate Alzheimer's, so as not to confuse them. Those with mild Alzheimer's will be well aware that it is December and that the group is planning a beach party. If you are just starting to work on a memory care unit, think about how to plan your activities ahead to actually coincide with an upcoming cultural or historical holiday, so that you are consciously working toward a theme event. For example, if you are starting the thematic programming in January, participants will know that Valentine's Day falls in February. Continuing with the garden theme, you can develop TTAP Method sessions based on a winter garden. Participants can be guided in creating centerpieces (step 4, sculpture) or colorful drawings and paintings (step 3, drawing the painting) for someone they love or a poem or short story about a special relationship (step 6, poetry, short stories). You can "build" up the activities to then be displayed and used during the theme event. The centerpieces can be used to decorate a table for a Valentine's Day party, the drawings and paintings can decorate the walls of the room where the event will take place, and each participant can share his or her poem or short story with everyone attending the event.

Theme events for individuals diagnosed with mild Alzheimer's can be quite fun. If you have just taken a new job in a facility, this is a great way to get your residents involved and create an awareness of your programs. Summertime offers many theme events (picnics, beach outings, movies, weddings). I have witnessed a couple living with mild Alzheimer's in a secured unit get married. The staff and residents decorated the day room, the kitchen prepared a large white cake, and the residents made flowers to throw at the happy couple. It was a lovely way to validate that at any age we can love, be loved, and share our love.

For those diagnosed in the moderate stages of Alzheimer's, you might not be able to link a number of weeks of programming together for an event that is a month away, but you can successfully start linking your TTAP programs together within a week or two of the event. Using the garden theme, the group conversation for step 1 can focus on Thanksgiving, or the Fall Harvest, a week or two before the actual holiday. For a group project, you can use a large canvas to create a colorful tablecloth (step 3, drawing and painting). Another adaptation would be to set up a large canvas the size of a table for four participants to sit around. The individuals would paint the portion of the canvas in front of them, and these decorative canvases would then be hung on the walls during the holiday celebration.

Developing a theme event for those with severe Alzheimer's could involve decorating the person's room with colored streamers on May Day, or bringing some paper objects in the form of a turkey or a pilgrim hat for the person to see and touch while encouraging a conversation with the person about Thanksgiving. The important element to remember in trying to engage someone with severe Alzheimer's in any of the steps of the TTAP Method is to continue your involvement; don't stop reaching out to the person, even if there is little to no response. There is still someone inside.

Theme events stimulate the sensory cortex (feeling) in the experiences of the event environment, the decorations created, and the memories stimulated. The occipital lobe (seeing) is stimulated by the external visualization of the event that the participants are witnessing and experiencing. The thought processes and release of endorphins in the mind and the body positively stimulate the reticular formation (arousal). The temporal lobe (hearing) is stimulated by the activities surrounding the party. While the participants interact with each other and share their individual insights, Broca's area (speech) is stimulated.

STEP 9. PHOTOTHERAPY

When working with clients who have Alzheimer's, the therapist must be prepared to accommodate the individuals' cognitive decline. Often, individuals need assistance accessing memories. Using photographs in thematic programming from the person's past or present as phototherapy is a great tool for stimulating memories.

The modern technologies of digital cameras, cell phones, and tablets such as the iPad® have revolutionized the taking and sharing of photographs. A picture can be taken and shared with others in a matter of minutes. Phototherapy, however, is not just about *taking* pictures; photographs are a powerful way to stimulate the recall of memories and to engage an individual in the process of life review. (See Chapter 2, "Photographs as Therapy in the TTAP Method," and Chapter 6, "Life Review and People with Alzheimer's Disease.")

Everyone has photographs that are important to them, that show the persons, places, and events that shaped who they are across the life span. Treasured photographs can be dynamic tools to engage individuals through the TTAP Method. In developing a phototherapy program the therapist should start by photocopying or scanning and printing photographs that belong to the group participants (of course, with their permission). The therapist can also take pictures of the participants themselves and reproduce those for use in a creative arts activity.

In the early stages of Alzheimer's there are many ways to use photographs through a thematic approach. I worked with a wonderful therapist, Beverly Forman, at The Hebrew Home for The Aged, in Riverdale, New York, to develop a phototherapy program for individuals with mild Alzheimer's. (Beverly passed away as I wrote this chapter, and I would like to dedicate this section on phototherapy to her

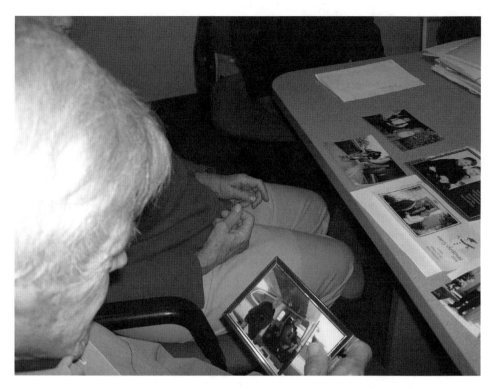

Figure 3.11.   Photographs, from the past or present, can stimulate the recall of memories for residents.

memory.) This was the first time I had used photographs in creative arts programming for individuals with Alzheimer's. The theme was womanhood, and the group we worked with was entirely made up of women. Each woman was asked to bring with her from her room photographs that were important to her. Beverly and I then copied the photographs in multiple colored images and then returned the originals to the women. Participants were each given an 18-by-24-inch poster board as well as glue and colored markers. They were directed to cut out the photographs and create a personal collage of all of the significant people in their lives. We also asked them to write down thoughts, stories, or memories about these people. Unbeknownst to Beverly and me, the group of 12 women worked on this project for over 4 weeks, meeting only once a week. (It is important to note here that thematic programming can be done as little or as often as desired within your daily activity schedule.) The final results were 12 poster boards hung up in the main hallway of the facility, each accompanied with a beautiful reflection of the people, places, and experiences that touched these women's lives. Beverly and I conducted a special celebration at the end of the phototherapy program, serving drinks and sweets and sharing each woman's story with the group.

Using photographs with those diagnosed with moderate Alzheimer's disease can also be very powerful. In a 2009 study of the use of the TTAP Method to stimulate cognitive functioning in people with moderate to severe Alzheimer's living in a skilled nursing facility at the Bergen Regional Medical Center in New Jersey, recreation therapists were allowed to make color photocopies of photographs borrowed, with permission, from the residents. The photocopies were used as part of a 7-week TTAP Method program along with original photographs that the residents brought with them. As part of the group conversation (step 1), the residents were asked to talk about their photographs (What do the photographs show? When were the photographs taken? Why are the photographs important to you? What memories do the photographs bring to mind?). Just this first step created a dynamic and powerful connection among the group members in reminiscing with each other. The residents were then given wooden picture frames and were asked to paint the frames however they chose. Glass mosaic tiles and other decorative pieces were also given to the residents and they were asked to paste whichever and however many of them onto their frames. When asked about their experience of the activity, resident responses included: "I never thought this activity could be so enjoyable"; "Remembering my family is important to me"; and "I enjoy listening to other peoples' lives."

Using phototherapy can also be a powerful experience for people with moderate to severe Alzheimer's. Old photographs can be enlarged and hung in the person's room to stimulate reminiscence. To enhance interactions, the therapist can ask questions about the places, persons, or experiences shown in the photographs. Residents can also be assisted in writing a love letter to someone shown in the picture, such as a grandchild.

Using photographs in creative arts programming stimulates the sensory cortex (feeling) in the reactions to what is being photographed. The occipital lobe (seeing) is stimulated by the visualization of the photographic process that participants are experiencing. The reticular formation (arousal) is positively stimulated by the thought processes and release of endorphins in the mind and the body. The temporal lobe (hearing) is stimulated by the group's conversations and the voice of the therapist. While the participants share their individual insights, Broca's area (speech) is being stimulated.

STEP 10. SENSORY STIMULATION

Sensory stimulation is probably the most powerful method in which to engage an individual, but especially those diagnosed with Alzheimer's. The senses can trigger multiple memories. When developing a sensory stimulation program, the therapist should first consult with facility staff regarding allergies or other specific sensitivities that a resident may have to oils, scents, or lotions.

Sensory stimulation offers many opportunities to engage those with mild Alzheimer's in thematic programming. Scents can represent any of the seasons. Floral scents, for example, can stimulate discussions of summer. The smell of pine or touching a pine cone can immediately bring to mind memories, stories, and images of wintertime. Seeing and touching fall leaves can elicit memories of childhood and time spent playing in piles of leaves in streets and backyards. Tree bark can be brought in and passed around for participants. Ask the group to close their eyes and feel the bark. What does it feel and smell like? What does it remind you of? These types of questions can lead to multiple conversations with and among your participants.

To stimulate the senses of those with moderate Alzheimer's, the therapist can bring in not only pine cones but also photographs of forests, pine scent oils, objects made from pine cones, and small pine cone trees. Try to heighten the visual, auditory, and sensory stimulation. The therapist could also bring in an enlarged famous painting, such as Monet's garden at Giverny, and have lily flowers, grass, and other beautiful objects that the participants might expect to find in a summer garden. Build on these sensory stimulating objects with conversations about people, places, and events of the past that participants recall and share with the group. A sensory stimulation program can grow naturally from a phototherapy, drawing/painting, or sculpture activity.

Sensory stimulation is one of the most important interactions for those with severe Alzheimer's. To best adapt a sensory program for this population, first learn as much as you can about the person's life story. Consider an activity a therapist shared with me. Her client lived on the island of Jamaica during her early life and had moved to the United States after becoming a mother. The woman was now bedridden, living in a skilled nursing facility and in the late stage of Alzheimer's. The therapist filled a shoe box full of sand and headed off to the client's room. She sat and spoke quietly with the woman, but her client would not respond and kept her eyes closed. The therapist slowly told the woman that she had brought her some sand to touch, that she might remember the sand from her family home as a child. The therapist slowly took the woman's hand and put it in the shoe box of sand. To her amazement, the woman opened her eyes and said, "I remember how my feet felt in the sand. I spent my childhood on the warm sandy beaches."

STEP 11. DRAMA OR THEATER EXPERIENCE

Theater, acting, and role-playing have become very popular as activities for those diagnosed with Alzheimer's. Objects or props, scripts, and personal stories can be transformed into plays and performances.

For those with mild Alzheimer's, begin the programming by asking the participants to share experiences from their past related to a theme (jobs, hobbies, travel). Document what they share and then use this information to guide your group to develop their personal stories into a play or theater show for others.

Using objects or props works well for those with moderate Alzheimer's to create impromptu drama activities. On a table place different hats representing all types of activities or jobs, such as a chef's hat, top hat, bonnet, straw hat, nurse's cap, or summer beach hat, then have your participants choose one of them. After each person chooses a hat, encourage him or her to take on the role the hat represents. You can start by asking "What would you say as this person in this hat?" or "What would your job be wearing this hat?" The therapist can direct these role-play interactions as a single group activity or on a weekly basis, building upon the interactions and growing them into a performance with each session.

Someone with severe Alzheimer's may still be able to respond to an object or prop. Think creatively of ways to stimulate your client using what you can learn of the person's life story. Bring in, for example, an object or prop the person may recall from his or her past. I worked once with a woman living in a long-term care unit who was very aggressive. Through her assessment I discovered that she had worked as a family physician in Spain. I brought in a stethoscope and gave it to the woman along with a baby doll. She immediately placed the scope around her neck and then on the baby doll's chest, as if to listen to its heartbeat. The woman became relaxed, and her aggressive behaviors were resolved through the use of a familiar object from her past.

STEP 12. CLIENT FEEDBACK, ASSESSMENT, AND EVALUATION

As a therapist, activity professional, or aide you must design your evaluation questions for feedback in very specific ways because each individual has both strengths and weaknesses. The last step of the TTAP

Method is significant in giving individuals with Alzheimer's a *voice* in the therapeutic programming. The ability to be heard is paramount to maintaining a sense of self. As discussed in Chapter 2, studies of the use of life review and reminiscence therapy for those diagnosed with Alzheimer's have shown that older adults want to achieve and maintain emotional well-being, especially in the face of significant physical or cognitive declines associated with advanced age or disease (Lee, Tabourne & Yoon, 2008). Feedback gathered during the two studies revealed six themes: The study participants wanted to feel connected through activities, to communicate with others, to be able to differentiate likes and dislikes and have choices, to express feelings and emotions, to have opportunities to recall memories, and to express emotions (Lee, Tabourne & Yoon, 2008). (See "The CCDERS Approach™ and the TTAP Method" in Chapter 2.)

Asking your participants how they enjoyed a program session and what they would like to do for future sessions is the basis of step 12. Client feedback, assessment, and evaluation also aid the therapist in measuring and documenting the effectiveness of each creative arts session. As discussed in detail in Chapter 7, efficacy in working with those diagnosed with Alzheimer's is paramount in relation to how creative arts programming can improve a client's treatment outcome, monetarily affects a facility, and increases opportunities for research. In today's society we need to justify, quantify, and measure the therapeutic goals and objectives we put forth.

The following questions can be used to gather feedback from the group participants following each programming session and can be adapted for those with mild or moderate Alzheimer's (adapted from the Farrington Leisure Questionnaire [American Therapeutic Recreation Association, 2008]). Ask each person to rate his or her response from 1 (lowest) to 5 (highest).

1. Did this activity make you feel bored at any time?

2. Are you looking forward to next week's session?

3. Did the meditation quiet your mind?

4. Were you in good spirits during this session?

5. Did this session take your mind off the future?

6. Did you feel restless or fidgety during this session?

7. Did this session help your memory?

8. Did this session add excitement to your life?

Asking these types of open-ended questions allows the therapist not only to document and demonstrate the effects of the programming sessions on the Alzheimer's population but also to validate each participant's experience of the creative arts activities, which will naturally enhance the individual's overall emotional well-being and quality of life.

INTERGENERATIONAL PROGRAMMING USING THE TTAP METHOD

As discussed in Chapter 2, family members, young and old, can play an essential role in engaging a loved one with Alzheimer's through conversation and interactions that stimulate responsiveness and verbalizations as the disease progresses. Research that has looked specifically at intergenerational programming (IGP) for older adults with dementia and children has found that children can play a dynamic role in the overall quality of life and psychosocial well-being of the adult participants. Consideration, of course, must be given to older adults' abilities and interests in developing and implementing beneficial IGP. Jarrott (2003) found that adults with a wide range of needs and abilities can successfully engage in IGP with children and that the programming itself is appropriate and effective for people with dementia. Jarrott also observed considerable levels of positive affect and behavioral engagement, specifically behaviors supporting personhood, and that the affect expressed by the adult participants was significantly higher when the children were present than when they were not, indicating a positive influence of joining the adults and children in activities.

The steps of the TTAP Method offer many opportunities for intergenerational programming. A word board or chart can be used with group conversation (step 1) to begin programming around discussion of a theme. One theme may be growth or change. The therapist gathers words, thoughts, and ideas from the older and younger group participants, focusing them on experiences of change and growth in their lives. Moving on next to a music and meditation exercise (step 2), the therapist can use music for a guided imagery, asking the participants to see something that has changed or grown in their lives. For the young people, they may see a younger sister or brother growing and changing, while the older adults will see their own personal experiences of growth and changes in their mind's eye. The pairs, guided by the therapist, can then go on to explore the chosen theme through the other steps of the TTAP Method.

For a drawing and painting activity (step 3), the therapist can hand out paper, pastels, and markers and ask the young person and older adult to draw a picture together of what they each saw in their mind's eye as part of the guided imagery exercise. A group writing experience (step 6) using the theme of change can begin by asking the pair to refer back to the word board or chart that was compiled for step 1 to write a story together about what it feels like to "witness changes." The two can be instructed to try to place the words into sentences, and to begin first by forming a title for their story on change. Or the therapist could instruct the pair to begin by having the child talk about his or her experiences of change from a child's perspective and then the older adult could share his or her experiences. Food programs (step 7) are always fun activities for the young and old to share. The therapist could have the pair write a list of their favorite foods, foods that changed from being their favorites to no longer their favorites, foods that change when cooked (hard to soft, dry to moist/wet, large to small, etc.), foods that change color when cooked, or foods that people eat with each change of season. The group could then pick a few good dishes that they can prepare together, creating an even more profound personal experience for the older adult and young person.

Creating a theme event intergenerationally can be fun and easy (step 8). Continuing with the theme of change or growth, the pair can use the list of foods from the food program to lead into a Thanksgiving celebration, maybe creating receipt books or stories of their favorite Thanksgiving dinners. The older adult can create the detailed recipes and the child can create a favorite story. On the actual day of the theme event, decorations that the group already created together (e.g., centerpiece sculptures [step 4], collages [step 3]), can be used to decorate the table and room. Remember to use a camera to document what fun the group had. After the event the therapist can use the photographs to lead into a phototherapy program (step 9). A photograph taken during the theme event can be given to each participant as well as a wooden frame to paint and decorate. The pair can then exchange the frame they created with the photograph inside. Color copies of photographs can also be handed out for the pair to use in creating a collage or photo album of the theme event. For a photo album, the pair can work together to create a cover, or the young person can make one cover and the older adult can make another. They can then work together to put the photographs in a book. The therapist can also have the pair write a sentence or two under each photograph, creating a storybook of the entire intergenerational experience.

Sensory stimulation can be incorporated into intergenerational programming in many ways (step 10). The therapist can provide different scented items (flowers, candles, perfumes/colognes) or small objects (pine cones, fruits, shells) to be used in challenges with other pairs in the group. The therapist can challenge the pairs to guess what the scent is or what the object is, and so forth. Or the therapist can provide one scent, such as the smell of pine cones, and ask each pair to write and speak about what the smell of pine cones brings to their mind's eye, or have them together sculpt their perfect pine cone (step 4), or together paint a pine cone in silver or gold (step 3) to use as a table centerpiece for a theme event (step 8), and so forth.

A drama or theater experience (step 11) can be used to set the stage for a play that the group has read together or is familiar with. The therapist and older adults can guide the younger participants in the roles they will be playing. This type of activity uses memory, cognition, and organizational skills of both the young people and older adults. The therapist can bring in props and objects for the pairs to choose from for whichever role each will choose to play or that the pair can use to create their own role-play performance based around the chosen theme.

For all intergenerational programming be sure to distribute a simple pre-activity questionnaire to the older adult participants, asking questions such as How do you think the program will affect you? Do you think you will feel differently after participating in the program? Do you look forward to starting the program? For the post-activity questionnaire, ask questions such as Did you enjoy the program (on a scale of 1 to 5, 1 being least enjoyed and 5 being most enjoyed)? What did you like the best? How did you feel after the program? As discussed in Chapter 7, feedback and evaluation are very important in documenting the success of intergenerational programming for participants with Alzheimer's and other dementias, and can be used when applying for funding for future programming. Remember the saying: If it's not written down, it didn't happen!

CONCLUSION

Applying the TTAP Method with people with Alzheimer's and other dementias has several benefits:

- Myriad opportunities are created for life review and reminiscence (incorporates past and present personal interests and life experiences) through the repeated and continual use of themes or objects, which is essential in delaying the progression of the disease by challenging the mind and stimulating positive changes in the brain.

- The strengths and abilities those with Alzheimer's can continue to possess during the course of the disease process are incorporated and promoted throughout the programming, including the ability to communicate and connect with others, differentiate likes and dislikes, express feelings and emotions, recall long-term memories, and self-express what they think and feel (Chapter 2, CCDERS Approach).

- Each participant's self-expression takes a central position in all programming.

- Through the repetitive stimulation of brain regions through a variety of programming, people with Alzheimer's can actively engage in purposeful and successful activities throughout the disease process.

- The combination of creative activities, social interactions, and opportunities for self-expression enhances self-esteem and intrinsic motivation for the older adult and encourages further participation in the programming.

- Each individual's unique combination of skills, interests, multiple intelligences, and capacity for self-expression is incorporated into all programming.

CHAPTER 4

Brain Functioning, Cognition, and the TTAP Method

Current research offers growing insight into not only how the brain functions but also how to stimulate different regions of the brain to improve its functioning. This chapter reviews studies on brain functioning and cognition as well as current research on Alzheimer's disease, brain physiology, memory and the brain, the effects of depression and stress on brain functioning and cognition, and the importance of early intervention in treating Alzheimer's. The TTAP Method® incorporates new knowledge of how the brain functions into a multimodal approach that integrates and stimulates different areas of the brain through a variety of therapeutic activities. New discoveries are opening the doors to new understandings of how the brain and its vast functions can be positively affected and influenced by a person's environments, actions, thoughts, and positive feelings about him- or herself throughout the disease process (Diamond, 2000; Levine Madori, 2007; Snowdon, 2001).

BRAIN RESEARCH

The 1990s were considered the decade of the brain because more was learned about brain function in that decade than ever before. Modern technology has enabled the discovery of new facts that have permanently altered previous concepts of how the brain functions. Child developmental research before 1990 subscribed to the belief that humans are born with a finite number of brain cells and that, throughout the life span, these cells slowly die off. This basic belief has been wholly disproved since the end of the 1990s.

The first attempts to understand the brain were made in the 1960s by a research team at the University of California, Berkeley. That research, conducted by Dr. Mark Rosenzweig and Dr. Marion Diamond, proved that the brain can make new cells when stimulated by visual, auditory, sensory, verbal, or kinesthetic stimuli (Diamond, 2000). The first research experiment divided a group of very young, genetically linked laboratory mice into two groups. The mice in one group were placed into much larger cages with visual and kinesthetic manipulative items, such as wheels, toys, and colorful objects, that were changed weekly to reinforce an enriched environment that encouraged the mice to experiment and interact daily with the new stimuli. The mice in the second group were placed in small cages without toys or other stimulation. After a year, both groups' brains were weighed, measured, and compared in size and mass. The findings proved, for the first time, a direct correlation between outside stimulation and brain mass and density. The mice with the enriched environment had increased brain mass and higher levels of neurotransmitters as a result of the constant cognitive stimulation. The mice that had received no external stimulation had decreased brain mass and significantly lower levels of neurotransmitters.

While the research at Berkeley progressed, new findings were being published by a research team at the University of Illinois. The research of Golomb et al. (1996) confirmed that cognitively active mice developed brains that were packed more densely with neurons. These mice also took less time to solve problems, such as learning how to find their way through a maze. The mice with no cognitive stimulation showed delayed responses and physical differences in brain mass.

In the continued research at Berkeley, Diamond (2000) showed for the first time biological evidence of the correlation between brain mass and density and lifestyle and education. Studies of 300 randomly donated brains revealed the existence of three distinct thicknesses in the cortical wall. Further investigation into the lifestyles of the people whose brains had been donated led to a significant scientific discovery: People with less than secondary education had the thinnest wall mass, those who had completed high school and then worked in unskilled jobs had the second thickest wall mass, and those who had completed high school and then gone on to higher education or technical positions had the most dense brain mass. Diamond (2000) concluded that even occupations that do not necessarily require higher education, such as carpentry, could result in thicker wall mass because of the continual thinking, choice making, and problem solving that are involved in these professions. Diamond's findings confirm that the brain is able to grow new cells and refute the previous belief that humans are born with a finite number of brain cells that slowly die off as one ages. This now-refuted notion underpins the common belief that age is related directly to senility.

Modern medicine, through technological breakthroughs, has also developed new understandings of the brain's ability to regrow cells in the hippocampus region, the area central to memory and learning. When the brain receives external stimulation, such as through reading, writing, and environmental cues, it causes the cells in this region to rejuvenate and reproduce. Such medical breakthroughs could affect dramatically how people understand the importance of therapeutic activities throughout the life span, as these activities relate to and directly affect brain wellness (Diamond, 2000). Therapists must incorporate this understanding into how they structure programming so that it better enhances cognitive functioning in the people they are assisting; that is, they must recognize the importance of continual sensory stimulation in all therapeutic programming.

The most significant later findings that support and complement those of earlier research come from a still-running longitudinal study begun in 1986 at the University of Kentucky: the Nun Study. David Snowdon has been studying 678 nuns, all of whom are members of a convent in Minnesota, since they were 16 years old (Lemonick & Park, 2001). All the nuns studied to become teachers. Their personal and medical histories have been researched, they have participated in testing of their cognitive abilities, and their brains have been studied after their deaths. In his book *Aging with Grace*, Snowdon (2001) revealed significant links between lifestyle in well older adults and the nuns who eventually developed senility, which today is known as Alzheimer's disease. Snowdon's findings show that a history of stroke or head trauma can increase the probability of developing some form of dementia or Alzheimer's, and that a college education and an active intellectual life may protect a person from the effects of dementia. The autobiographical information written by the nuns was studied for detail, expression of thought, and complexity of idea. One surprising finding, according to Snowdon, is that "the way we express ourselves in language, even at an early age, can foretell how long we'll live and how vulnerable we are to getting the disease decades down the line."

In 2006, Dr. Richard Faull and his colleagues at the University of Auckland in New Zealand were the first to photograph the hippocampus region having regrown cells in individuals in their late 80s and early 90s. Dr. Faull and his colleagues won the Nobel Prize in 2008 for this scientific discovery. Faull's research adds to the body of knowledge continuing to prove scientifically that the brain can repair itself to some degree. A 5-year study published in 2006 on the long-term effects of cognitive training on everyday functional outcomes in older adults provided more evidence of the ability to reverse brain atrophy and thereby improve cognition. The study, which was conducted between April 1998 and December 2004, followed 2,832 people (ages 75 to 80) from six U.S. cities who were recruited from senior housing, community centers, and hospitals. All participants received sessions for memory (verbal episodic memory), reasoning (inductive reasoning), or speed of processing (visual search and identification). Performance-based measures and self-reporting indicated significantly less difficulty in the activities of daily living, improved reasoning, and an increase in the speed of processing. The cognitive scales showed a positive and significant correlation to increased cognitive abilities and overall quality of life over the 5-year period (Willis et al., 2006).

These research findings aid in assembling the puzzle pieces of how the mind works. At the core of the findings is the realization that the more stimulation the brain receives, the better it functions. Providing better programming that incorporates and fosters brain stimulation through social, verbal, visual, and auditory activities is essential for enhancing brain functioning and cognition. If brain cells regrow when brain stimulation occurs, then this stimulation could conceivably contribute to a delay in the progression of Alzheimer's, which if true can directly affect the quality of life of people with the disease. (Chapter 5, Using the TTAP Method to Stimulate Brain Functioning, discusses how each step in the TTAP Method works and what parts of the brain are consequently stimulated.)

BRAIN REGIONS

Figure 4.1 shows the different areas of the brain, each of which controls specific body functions as well as different perceptions and senses. The following is a description of each of the areas:

> *Cerebrum:* The largest and most highly developed part of the human brain, the cerebrum encompasses about two-thirds of the brain and is divided into right and left hemispheres that in turn are divided into four *lobes* (*frontal, parietal, occipital,* and *temporal*).

> *Cerebral cortex:* A thin layer of tissue that covers the outermost layer of the cerebrum. Together, the cerebral cortex and the cerebrum are the largest part of the human brain, associated with higher brain function, such as consciousness. (See Figure 4.2.)

> *Neocortex:* Occupying the bulk of the cerebrum and cerebral cortex, the neocortex is divided into four *lobes:*

> > *–Frontal lobe:* This region is future oriented and functions both creatively and analytically. To the right, the functions are artistic and creative. To the left is the analytical part of the brain, which deals with problem solving and complex

math. The frontal lobe also helps determine the complexity of one's personality.

–*Parietal lobe:* Located at the top of the brain, this area is associated with the sense of touch and also senses hot and cold, hard and soft, degrees of pain, and taste and smell.

–*Occipital lobe:* Located in the back of the brain, this area controls vision and discerns shapes, colors, and movements.

–*Temporal lobe:* The center for hearing and auditory processing, the temporal lobe receives auditory signals and identifies sounds by comparing them with sound patterns stored in memory.

Motor cortex: One of the primary regions of the neocortex in the frontal lobe, this area governs movement and overall motor control. Many motor defects can take place in this region.

Sensory cortex: Located in the parietal lobe, this area involves taste and smell and is commonly affected by brain injury or trauma; the person often loses his or her sense of smell or taste.

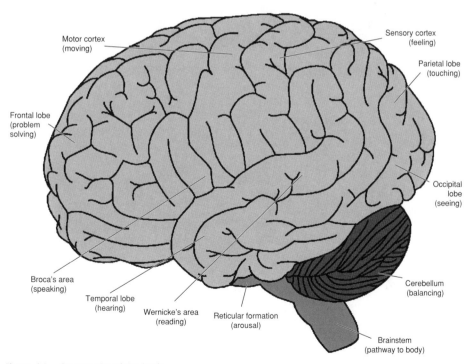

Figure 4.1.   Geography of the brain.

A

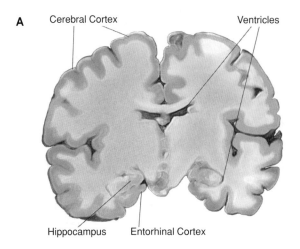

B

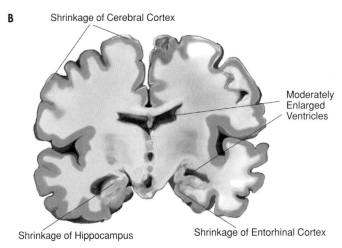

C

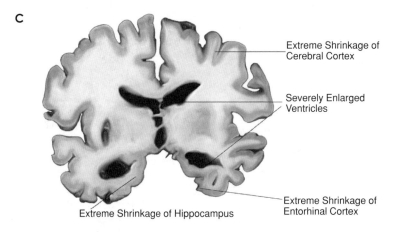

Figure 4.2 (A, B, C).   Shrinkage of the cerebral cortex, hippocampus, and entorhinal cortex during the progression of Alzheimer's disease (*A*, preclinical Alzheimer's; *B*, mild to moderate Alzheimer's; and *C*, severe Alzheimer's). (Images courtesy of the National Institute on Aging/National Institutes of Health.)

Wernicke's area: Located in the cerebral cortex where the temporal and parietal lobes meet, this area is the center for understanding written and spoken language.

Broca's area: Located in the frontal lobe, this area is responsible for speech, including the control of motor functions involved in speech production.

Cerebellum: Located in the back of the brain, this area is the center of balance for the body. It coordinates movement as it monitors impulses from nerve endings in the muscles.

Brain stem: Located at the base of the brain and extending over the spinal column, the brain stem is the brain path to the body. It is the center for sensory reception, and it monitors vital bodily functions, including heartbeat, breathing, and digestion.

Reticular formation: Located between the brain stem and extending to the spinal column, this region is the trigger area for arousal. The reticular formation acts as a chemical crossover for neurons that opens and closes with stimulation from sex, drugs, or food. Studies have shown that the reticular formation is one of the last regions of the brain to be affected by the abnormal plaques and tangles of Alzheimer's (Ishii, 2004).

Hippocampus: Located in the temporal lobe, this area of the brain forms complex memories. (See Figure 4.2.)

Entorhinal cortex: Part of the temporal lobe near the hippocampus, this is a memory-processing center that is involved in the formation and consolidation of memories. It also serves as the main conduit for translating information between the hippocampus and neocortex. Studies indicate that the accumulation of beta amyloid plaques and tangles associated with mild to moderate Alzheimer's and the decline in cognitive performance begin in this area (Arehart-Treichel, 2001; Ishii, 2004; Thompson, 2003). (See Figure 4.2.)

Figure 4.2 shows the regions of the brain that are slowly destroyed during the progression of Alzheimer's, specifically the cerebral cortex, hippocampus, and entorhinal cortex. In the first stage of the disease, the area affected is the entorhinal cortex, the memory-processing center essential for making new memories and retrieving short-term memories. This stage can last from 1 to 9 years. In the second stage, the plaques and tangles move higher, invading the hippocampus, the part of the brain that forms complex memories. This stage can last from

2 to 5 years. In the third stage, which can last from 1 to 3 years, the plaques and tangles reach the top of the brain, known as the neocortex or the "executive region," which sorts through stimuli and orchestrates all behavior and higher brain functioning across the four lobes.

MEMORY AND THE BRAIN

It has been hypothesized that memory processing at the neuronal level of the hippocampus takes place only in the presence of the neurotransmitter acetylcholine. (*Neurotransmitters* transmit signals from a neuron to a target cell across a synapse.) Coghill (2000) found a decrease in the amounts of acetylcholine in the temporal lobe of people who showed symptoms of memory loss. Therefore, with cerebral cell loss and a decrease in the amount of acetylcholine in and around the hippocampus as a result of the aging of the brain, people experience loss of memory, and their memory functions are dramatically compromised. According to the *Diagnostic and Statistical Manual of Mental Disorders* (DSM-IV; American Psychiatric Association, 2000), the essential feature in the syndrome of all dementias is a significant enough loss of intellectual abilities to interfere with social or occupational functioning. The deficit is multifaceted and can involve memory, judgment, abstract thinking, thought processes, and a variety of other higher cortical functions. Changes in personality and behavior also occur.

The Latria–Nebraska Neuropsychological Battery (LNNB) was developed to help therapists of various disciplines identify the remaining skills of an individual with Alzheimer's (Barrett, 1986). The premise behind the LNNB is that the brain operates as a whole, yet each section seems to provide a separate function. Many higher-level functions depend on a variety of similar skills. The pathological processes of the beta amyloid proteins that produce the plaques and tangles of dementia can progress slowly as they travel through the brain. If we can compensate for the person's brain functions through areas that are still intact, we might be able to develop new systems for structural change in the brain by assessing, planning, and implementing therapeutic interventions. Thus, identifying the remaining skills helps to establish alternative functions.

Barrett (1986) addressed the significance of this revelation regarding brain functioning in the case of dementia, noting that repetitive stimulation of existing cell structures in the neocortex, such as the repetition of previously learned behaviors (e.g., using fine motor coordination to knit or type), could facilitate the recall of memories and other learned behaviors. This understanding of how to stimulate the brain to retrieve old memories strongly relates to reframing the role of therapeutic activities in relation to cognitive deterioration or early-onset Alzheimer's (Stern, Albert, Tang, & Tsai, 1999; Stern et al., 1994; Stern, Moeller, & Anderson, 2000). Therapists need to focus on the stimulation that takes place during therapeutic interventions and on what areas of the brain are affected. (See Chapter 5.)

NEUROPLASTICITY AND COGNITIVE RESERVE

Neuroplasticity (or *brain plasticity*) is the brain's ability to retain new information and create new ideas throughout the life span in response to learning (Finnemore, 2009). Although it is true that we lose thousands of brain cells each day, studies have shown that individuals continue to grow new cells throughout life in response to influences and experiences as they age (Nelson, 2005). As mentioned earlier, sensory stimulation can be used to target specific regions to create more mass and density, a phenomenon known as *cognitive reserve*. Research on neuroplasticity and cognitive reserve holds great promise in developing interventions to slow the progression of early-stage dementia or Alzheimer's.

For example, a 2007 study of neuroplasticity examined mice that had been bred to develop the plaques and tangles characteristic of Alzheimer's and found a direct link between learning and enhanced cell regrowth in the brain (LaFerla, McGaugh, Green, & Billings, 2007). The researchers studied hundreds of these specially bred mice between the ages of 2 and 18 months. Mice in one group were allowed to learn by swimming in a round tank of water until they found a submerged platform on which to stand. These mice received training four times a day for 1 week at 2, 6, 9, 12, 15, and 18 months of age and were evaluated at each session for learning and memory abilities. Other groups of untrained mice were allowed to swim in the tank for just one session before testing their learning and memory skills and examining their brains for plaques and tangles. Mice up to 12 months of age that learned on previous occasions had fewer plaques and tangles in their brains, and they learned and remembered the location of the escape platform much better than mice not previously allowed to learn. At the 12-month point, the mice that had learned developed levels of beta amyloid that were 60% less than those of the mice that had not learned. By 15 months of age, however, the mice that had learned deteriorated and were identical both physically and cognitively to the mice that had not learned. "We were surprised this mild learning had such big effects at reducing Alzheimer's disease pathology and cognitive decline, but the effects were not strong enough to overcome later and more severe pathology," Green reported. "We are now investigating if more frequent and vigorous learning will have bigger and longer benefits to Alzheimer's disease."

CURRENT RESEARCH ON ALZHEIMER'S DISEASE

The aging population is currently the largest cohort in U.S. history. Between 2000 and 2010, the number of adults age 65 or older increased at a faster rate (15.1%) than the total U.S. population (9.7%) (U.S. Census Bureau, 2011). Older adults comprise 13% of the total U.S. population, or 40.3 million people. It is estimated that by 2050, 20% of the U.S. population will be age 60 or older, or 88.5 million people. The prevalence of mild cognitive impairment (MCI) in the general population is reported at 10%–20% for adults age 65 and older, but is more common among people age 75 and older (Kumara et al., 2005; Manly, Tang, Schupf, & Stern, 2005; Ofstedal et al., 2007; Alzheimer's Association, 2011). The progression from MCI to Alzheimer's disease per year is reported to be roughly 15% (Davie et al., 2004; Fernandez-Ballesteros, Zamarron, Tarraga, Moya, & Iniguez, 2003; Alzheimer's Association, 2011). Some people, however, do not progress to a diagnosis of dementia, and they have the potential to improve cognition and memory with early interventions (Kluger, Ferris, Golomb, Mittelman, & Reisberg, 1999; Kramer et al., 2004).

Studies focused on psychosocial interventions have demonstrated that people with MCI or early-stage Alzheimer's have specific social, emotional, cognitive, and physical needs (Cotrell & Schulty, 1993; Garand, Buckwalter, & Hall, 2000; Gilley et al., 2004). Evidence suggests that activities in the cognitive, physical, and social domains help protect against cognitive decline and the onset of dementia (Burgener & Dickson-Putman, 1999). More specifically, continued active participation in life through interpersonal interactions and social activities that are individualized and person centered to each individual's needs and skills has been documented to enhance feelings of self-esteem and to directly improve overall quality of life (Pruessner et al., 2004). A national study of all research related to early-stage MCI or dementia indicated that psychosocial support for people newly diagnosed should be initiated soon after the diagnosis to prevent the person from falling into a pattern of self-isolation and dropping social support networks, which can speed cognitive decline and increase institutionalization rates (Fratiglioni, Paillard-Borg, & Winblad, 2004).

In a landmark study, Braak and Braak (1997) examined the most significant physical characteristics of Alzheimer's—beta amyloid plaques and tangles. The study of 2,261 brains on autopsy of people who had Alzheimer's allowed Braak and Braak to identify six related stages (I–VI) of change in the growth of the plaques and tangles during the progression of the disease. As a person progresses through the mild, moderate, and severe stages of the disease, the plaques and tangles grow simultaneously. In Stage I, early changes in the number of plaques and tangles are restricted to the entorhinal cortex. In Stages II and III, the plaques and tangles travel beyond the entorhinal cortex, invading the hippocampus region. In the final three stages, Stages IV to VI, more global dysfunction becomes evident with the progression of the plaques and tangles to the temporal and frontal lobes of the neocortex. Previous Alzheimer's researchers had noted brain deterioration and impairment in brain functioning with attendant cognitive deficits but were unclear about their origins (Reisberg, Ferris, de Leon, & Crook, 1982). It was not until Braak and Braak (1997) discovered that a greater number of plaques and tangles correlated with a greater deterioration of brain cells that the etiology of Alzheimer's, with its concomitant impairments in behavioral and cognitive functioning, became clearer. The location of brain abnormalities and their relationship to brain functioning, specifically regarding cognitive functioning, is significant in understanding and attempting to delay the progression of Alzheimer's. The University of California, Los Angeles (UCLA) and the University of Queensland (Australia) published videos using magnetic resonance imaging (MRI) that made it possible to "see" into the brain and observe the wave of tissue loss as the plaques and tangles move across the brain to the executive region, similar to the flow of lava (Thompson, 2003). Thompson's findings corresponded to those of Braak and Braak's (1997) autopsy research. This discovery of the specific pathway of the beta amyloid plaques and tangles became a momentous breakthrough. Namely, if cognitive, social, and physical stimulation can improve the brain's cell reserve in the hippocampus region, then the progression of Alzheimer's can be slowed (Diamond, 2000; Golomb et al., 1996; McClellen, 2001; Snowdon, 2001).

Weekly stimulation of communication and language in those affected by Alzheimer's has been proven valuable not only in delaying the progress of the disease but also in improving some cognitive functions. In a study published in a 2004 issue of the *Brazilian Journal of Medical and Biological Research*, nonpharmacological strategies, such as conversation, memory, and learning activities, were given to five older adults diagnosed with Alzheimer's. Findings showed that weekly stimulation of memory through language activities proved to be an effective intervention. Although the study specifically addressed neuropsychological rehabilitation, which is used to treat patients who have sustained cognitive, emotional, and behavioral impairments as the result of a brain injury, the data suggest that patients are able to preserve, maintain, and in some cases improve their cognitive functioning abilities by engaging in activities that stimulate language and communication (Fratiglioni et al., 2004; Hebert et al., 2000; Ryan, 2006).

Figure 4.2A shows the proximity of the entorhinal cortex and hippocampus region. In a 2-year study of older adults with Alzheimer's and those without, results demonstrated that the hippocampus region changes more drastically in both mass and density when invaded by the abnormal plaques and tangles of the disease. The volume of the hippocampus decreased about 4% over the 2-year period in older adults without the disease. For people who had been diagnosed with Alzheimer's, the volume decreased by 10% in the 2-year period. Evidence that the entorhinal cortex is the first brain area to deteriorate with Alzheimer's was first presented by Dr. Mony de Leon at the World Alzheimer's Congress in 2000. De Leon and his team of neuroscientists used MRIs and computed axial tomography (CAT) scans to study 48 people with normal cognition over a 3-year period (de Leon et al., 2001). His study sought to identify exactly what areas of the brain are affected by the disease and in what order. Over the 3-year period, 11 of the 48 subjects were diagnosed with Alzheimer's. Each of the 11 was initially shown to have lower glucose metabolism in the region of the entorhinal cortex in comparison to the other subjects. At the end of the 3-year study period, all 11 had signs of low glucose metabolism in the entorhinal cortex and in the hippocampus region. Thus the study further confirms the relationship between the deterioration in size, mass, and density of the entorhinal cortex and the hippocampus region and the disease process.

The frontal lobes are considered home to all of our likes and dislikes (essentially our personality traits), as well as the ability to solve problems. Other important functions lie in the frontal lobe, including motor coordination, spontaneity, being in the moment, memory, language, initiative, judgment, impulse control, and social and sexual behaviors. When a person is interacting one-on-one with a friend or loved one, reminiscing about the past, or is in a creative group experience deciding what colors to use to paint with, the frontal lobe region of the brain is directly affected by this stimulation, interaction, and self-expression (Levine Madori, 2007).

Both Broca's area and Wernicke's area are stimulated by conversation and language use. Studies have correlated the rich use of language (sessions designed to stimulate verbal memory) and reasoning (inductive reasoning through problem solving) with increased cognition and improved reasoning skills and processing speed (Willis et al., 2006).

The cerebellum is a relatively neglected area and underaddressed in research on Alzheimer's disease. It was previously thought that the disease spares this region. Researchers, however, have since proven—primarily by studying brain tissue—that a number of pathological changes take place in the cerebellum of people with Alzheimer's. Abnormal beta amyloid proteins have been found, but not the tangles closely correlated with the disease process. For this reason, the use of sensory stimulation (seeing, hearing, touch, smell, and taste) throughout the disease process is recommended in an effort to protect this region of the brain and capitalize on its latent capabilities (Larner, 1997).

DEPRESSION, EMOTIONS, AND COGNITION

Cognitive evaluations have shown significantly impaired performance during depressive states (Butters, Becker, Nebes, Zmuda, Mulsant, & Pollock, 2000; Gray, Braver, & Raichle, 2002; Steffens et al., 2006; Tarbuck & Paykel, 1995). Clinically significant levels of depressive symptoms are found in 15%–30% of people with Alzheimer's, although they do not meet diagnostic criteria for major depression. Additionally, after age 70, the combination of impaired cognitive and depressive symptoms doubles in frequency every 5 years (Gilley et al., 2004). A 4-year longitudinal study evaluated contributing factors related to the development of progressive symptoms of depression in 410 people with Alzheimer's (Gilley et al., 2004). Researchers found that people between the ages of 45 and 65 with the disease had more intense depressive symptoms. Depression is treatable, and these findings support the need to assess people with early-stage Alzheimer's to help them maximize, retain, or regain their abilities. Successfully treating depression in older adults has been correlated with significantly alleviating cognitive impairments (Frazer, Christensen, & Griffiths, 2005). Research findings further demonstrate that treatment programs should have the capacity to enhance mood to elevate the client's perceived level of health and well-being.

Emotional states can also affect cognition. For example, anxiety is common in late life and has been proven to impair cognitive functioning in older adults (Beurs et al., 1999). Using functional MRIs, researchers have shown that emotional states, such as anxiety, affect cognition by modulating neural activity in the lateral prefrontal cortex (Gray et al., 2002). Adults are able to regulate their emotions by changing the way they conceptualize and experience everyday life challenges. Findings, however, suggest that some forms of emotional regulation may negatively affect cognitive functioning. One example is concealing outward signs of emotion. A person who withdraws emotionally is repressing the essence of him- or herself. Such repression has been linked with degraded memory, communication, and problem solving (Snowdon, 2001).

STRESS AND COGNITION

Numerous studies have documented the effects of stress on the body. Stress can raise a person's blood pressure, weaken the immune system, raise resting heart rate, and make someone feel nervous or faint. People can also experience tightness in their shoulders or neck area and have shallow breathing, headaches, stomachaches, or general pain. Some people feel overly tired when they are stressed, whereas others feel energetic or jittery. Too much stress can affect cognitive and emotional health. You may have trouble focusing, have difficulty making everyday decisions, or feel depressed or helpless. Some people may view and treat themselves negatively in response to stress and may have difficulty enjoying their usual interests.

Researchers have found that short- and long-term stress can negatively affect cognition and memory. According to a study conducted by Latham (2007), stress that lasts as little as a few hours can impair brain cell communication in areas associated with learning and memory. The study also found that acute, long-term stress activates molecules that impair the memory collection and storage processes in the brain. According to a study reported by the University of California, Irvine (2007), stress causes stress hormones in the brain to divert energy from the hippocampus (the area of the brain that is central to learning and memory) to areas that need it more. This decrease in available energy compromises the brain's ability to create new memories or to recall existing memories.

A diagnosis of Alzheimer's disease can cause immediate stress for the person diagnosed and, as mentioned earlier, may cause him or her to fall into a pattern of self-isolation (disengaging in social support networks), which can speed cognitive decline and lead to increased institutionalization rates. Researchers believe that treatments to slow or stop the progression of Alzheimer's disease and preserve cognitive function will be most effective when administered early in the course of the disease.

IMPORTANCE OF EARLY INTERVENTION
FOR PEOPLE WITH ALZHEIMER'S DISEASE

Why is early intervention crucial? Scientists know that the effects of the progression of Alzheimer's on life span depend specifically on the age when a person is first diagnosed. The median survival could range from nearly 9 years for people diagnosed at age 65 to approximately 3 years for those diagnosed at age 90. For those diagnosed in their 60s and early 70s, caregivers, patients, and their families can plan on a median life span of 7–20 years following the diagnosis. Emotional support, stimulating communication, and enriching experiences that provide the person with intrinsic motivation are important following a diagnosis of Alzheimer's disease. The sooner an individual is engaged in cognitively challenging activities, such as those that can be structured using the TTAP Method, the longer and healthier his or her life will be (Brookmeyer, Corrada, Curriero, & Kawas, 2002; Levine Madori, 2009a, 2009b, 2009c; Alders & Levine Madori, 2010).

For a person at any stage of the Alzheimer's disease process, memory losses can strongly affect self-confidence and can lead to anxiety, stress, depression, and withdrawal from activities. Withdrawal can result in a general increase in symptoms, including memory loss. This increase in symptoms beyond those directly attributable to the disease processes in the brain is an example of what has been called *excess disability* (Reifler & Larson, 1990). Early interventions can optimize memory and recall as well as assist in finding ways to compensate for abilities and skills that have been lost. Therapists and other caregivers can enhance remaining abilities by identifying the best ways of incorporating information that is meaningful to a person with Alzheimer's into daily therapeutic art and recreation.

CONCLUSION

When a person receives a diagnosis of Alzheimer's disease, the news is immediately accompanied by deep feelings of loss. This loss has been described as a loss of control, a loss of one's thoughts, and, probably most profoundly, a loss of self (i.e., cognitive functioning, skills and abilities, and expression of likes and dislikes). Thoughts such as "What will happen to me?" and "When will I start losing my mind?" are some of the first natural responses. Then the mind moves to the next natural psychological response, which is "What can I do?" Until now, the only response to this question was from a physician offering a prescription for medication that "might or might not help."

Current brain research continues to show that more varied interventions may exist that offer richer results. We *can* change the chemistry and physiology of the brain by actively and meaningfully engaging those with Alzheimer's. Therapists need to focus on the stimulation that takes place during therapeutic interventions and understand what areas of the brain are affected. Only then can targeted interventions be developed to enhance the brain's own ability to slow the progression of Alzheimer's.

As will be discussed in the next chapter, the TTAP Method uses the creative arts to link each session to specific areas of brain function.

Through the TTAP Method, participants are continually engaged in conversation that incorporates past and present personal interests and lifelong pursuits. Although more research is needed, the verbal, visual, social, and cognitive stimulation fostered through use of the TTAP Method might be proven to slow or alter the course of Alzheimer's. The TTAP Method uses dynamic interaction by incorporating avenues for both verbal and nonverbal communication in a group context, which has been shown to regulate functions in the cerebral cortex, thereby promoting brain wellness and skill retention among older adults (Claire et al., 2004; Diamond, 2000; Hass-Cohen & Carr, 2008; Kramer et al., 2004; McKinney, Antoni, Kumar, Tims, & McCabe, 1997).

CHAPTER 5

Using the TTAP Method to Stimulate Cognitive Functioning

As discussed in Chapter 4, research on brain functioning, brain plasticity, and cognitive reserve demonstrates that positive changes in cognition can be achieved through visual, verbal, and social stimulation. The TTAP Method® incorporates this information into a therapeutic approach for people with Alzheimer's disease that stimulates different regions of the brain through a variety of creative arts activities. This chapter explains the foundations of the TTAP Method in relation to current research on learning and intelligence as well as cognitive stimulation. Theories of how people process and store information are presented in relation to Benjamin Bloom's six levels of learning and Howard Gardner's seven learning styles. The chapter also explains the essential roles that emotions, imagination, and creativity play in stimulating the brain. Finally, an appendix to this chapter presents a 2009 study of the use of the TTAP Method to stimulate cognitive functioning in people with moderate to severe Alzheimer's living in a skilled nursing facility at the Bergen Regional Medical Center in New Jersey.

LEARNING AND INTELLIGENCE

It is hard to imagine that despite the same brain structures, every individual is different. Therapists ponder this every day as they look to the next new client or assessment. The notion that humans all have different frames of mind and multiple ways of using their intellect took a century to establish by cognitive developmentalists, such as Benjamin Bloom and Howard Gardner.

Benjamin Bloom

In 1956, Benjamin Bloom chaired a committee of educators who developed a classification of student learning objectives. Published as *Bloom's Taxonomy*, the committee's proposals represented an innovative approach to understanding the differences in learning (Bloom, 1956).

The theory was accepted across the United States in educational systems, giving rise to a new way to teach children so that they can learn better how to process new information. Bloom broke down the process of how we learn into six levels: knowledge, comprehension, application, analysis, synthesis, and evaluation.

Knowledge.   Knowledge is the recall of previously learned material. In the early 1950s, students typically were taught using memorization of charts and tables. In Bloom's theory, knowledge is the lowest level of learning, because facts and figures are regurgitated without any real understanding of their meaning. For example, a cashier gives change from a purchase simply by following the numbers on the cash register without calculating the difference between the amount that the customer gives and the amount of the purchase.

Comprehension.   Comprehension is the ability to capture the meaning of the information. The interpretation of information by explanation or summarization demonstrates that the learning process has moved beyond the simple memorization of material, according to Bloom. This can be demonstrated by changing the material from one form to another. For example, comprehension is the understanding of the translation of words and descriptions into mathematical figures (e.g., asking a person to represent what 7/8 of the whole is by using a pie cut up into 8 slices).

Application.   Application is the ability to use learned information in separate and distinct situations. This could include using the rules, principles, and laws of one area in another. An example of this stage of learning is applying learned information and using it in a new or unique way (e.g., how can you locate the post office in an unfamiliar city?). Understanding and applying methods of problem solving is a higher level of learning than comprehension.

Analysis.   Analysis is the ability to break down material into components or parts so that its pattern is understood. This includes the identification of the parts, analysis of the relationships between parts, and understanding of structural principles. Analysis is a higher intellectual level than comprehension and involves the ability to categorize the information one has learned. Once the information has been categorized, it then can be dissected from the whole to understand its meaning. An example would be understanding the various skills that contribute to a person's ability to put work aside and go for a weekend vacation.

Synthesis.   Synthesis is the ability to put together parts to form a new whole. This involves a unique understanding of the information and a plan of operation. Synthesis is the ability to use all that has been learned through knowledge, comprehension, application, and analysis to create a new or unique way of understanding that leads to connecting concepts into new patterns or structures. For example, a medical engineer uses knowledge from the field of physics in developing a new medical tool for laser surgery.

Evaluation.   Evaluation is the ability to judge the value of the process. The judgments are objective or subjective and based on specific, defined criteria, which may be internal (organization) or external (relevant to the purpose). Evaluation is the highest cognitive level because it encompasses all other levels. A cook who tries a new recipe and decides she will use more or less of an ingredient the next time it is prepared is using her powers of evaluation.

Howard Gardner

The work of Harvard psychologist Howard Gardner emerged in the early 1980s. Gardner's theory on learning, a culmination of his many years of research in cognitive psychology and neuropsychology, draws not only from Bloom, but also from the findings from more recent studies showing that the brain has multiple forms of intelligence, which can be stimulated by the way in which one is taught.

During his research, Gardner spent the mornings at a trauma and brain injury unit at Boston University Aphasic Research Center, where he focused on how the brain malfunctioned as a result of an injury, and in the afternoons he went to his other laboratory at Harvard's Project Zero, where he worked closely with gifted and talented children to understand the development of human cognitive capacities. By researching brain incapacitation, Gardner discovered and documented which areas of the brain were responsible for various functions. Gardner (1997) then applied what he had learned in these two converse settings to develop the concept of *seven styles of learning*, or *multiple intelligences*, in which he explains that different people learn in different ways.

Table 5.1 describes the seven distinct learning styles: *linguistic learner*, or word player; *logical learner*, or questioner; *spatial learner*, or visualizer; *musical learner*, or music lover; *kinesthetic learner*, or mover; *interpersonal learner*, or socializer; and *intrapersonal learner*, or individual. In the TTAP Method, each session of the creative arts programming is structured around these distinct learning styles to ensure that every individual learning style is incorporated into the therapeutic environment. Many learning styles can be incorporated into one experience. The primary goal of a good therapist is to adapt each session to

Table 5.1. Gardner's seven styles of learners

Type	Likes to	Is good at	Learns best
Linguistic learner (the word player)	Read, write, tell stories	Memorizing names, places, dates, trivia	Saying and hearing, seeing and visualizing
Logical learner (the questioner)	Do experiments, figure things out, explore patterns and relationships	Math, reasoning, logic, problem solving	Categorizing, classifying, working with abstract patterning
Spatial learner (the visualizer)	Draw, build, design, daydream, look at pictures, watch movies, play with machines	Imagining things, sensing changes, puzzles, reading maps, charting	Visualizing, dreaming, using the mind's eye, working with color
Musical learner (the music lover)	Sing, hum tunes, play an instrument, respond to music	Picking up sounds, remembering melodies, noticing pitches, keeping time	Rhythm, melody, music
Kinesthetic learner (the mover)	Move around, touch and talk, use body language	Physical activities (sports, dance, acting, crafts)	Touching, moving, interacting with space, processing knowledge through body sensations
Interpersonal learner (the socializer)	Have lots of friends, talk to people, join groups	Understanding people, leading others, organizing, communication, mediating conflicts	Sharing, comparing, relating, cooperating, interviewing
Intrapersonal learner (the individual)	Work alone, pursue own interests separately	Understanding self, focusing inward, following instincts, pursuing interests	Working alone, individual projects, self-paced/having own space

From Gardner, H. (1997). *Extraordinary minds: Portraits of exceptional individuals and an examination of our extraordinariness.* New York: Basic Books.

all levels of individual functioning within the group. This is one of the most complex tasks for therapists, yet they are rarely trained to handle these situations. The therapist can best meet the needs of each client with Alzheimer's by first assessing which of Gardner's seven learning styles he or she uses. (See the TTAP Method Activity Assessment form in Appendix B.)

Learning and Perception Using Three Brain Systems

Gardner took Bloom's understanding of learning one step further by defining the brain as having three systems of learning. These systems can be applied to understanding how the brain takes in, processes, and retrieves information. Using the locations and functions of the brain, Gardner collapsed Bloom's six styles of learning into three unique systems that can be incorporated in and used as a structure and foun-

Box 5.1. Gardner's three systems of learning

Affective system: Cortical, Subcortical lobes

- Limbic systems
- Happiness and fear
- All patterns of emotions

Strategic system: Interior, Frontal lobes

- Speaking and reading
- Fine motor skills, use of fingers
- Planning and the ability to mentally organize

Recognition system: Occipital, Parietal, Temporal lobes

- Recognition of faces and voices
- Matching of objects with sounds
- Identification of patterns

dation for therapeutic programming. Gardner identified the three systems as *affective, strategic,* and *recognition* (Box 5.1). The affective system lies in the cortical and subcortical regions, which is also where the limbic system resides. This system is described as the seat of emotions, ranging from fear to great happiness. The strategic system is located in the interior and frontal lobes and involves planning, fine motor skills, speaking, and reading. The recognition system is located in the occipital, parietal, and temporal lobes and is responsible for identifying patterns, which can be letters and words. It is also responsible for identifying faces and voices that are familiar or unfamiliar.

COGNITIVE STIMULATION AND THEMATIC PROGRAMMING

In addition to being grounded in cognitive psychology and neuropsychology, Gardner's theory of multiple intelligences also has a biological basis that has been proven through modern technology. As discussed in Chapter 3, certain cognitive functions can be tied to specific brain regions, as seen through CAT, PET, and MRI imaging and as evidenced by the loss of certain cognitive functioning as a result of brain injury. This premise takes into account the brain as a major physical determinant of intelligence (Li, 1996). By studying people who had a speech impairment, who were paralyzed, or who had other disabilities, Gardner identified the parts of the brain that were needed to perform certain cognitive and physical functions. He then related each learning style to a specific region of the brain. This same biological basis corre-

Table 5.2.   Steps of the TTAP Method related to learning styles used and brain region(s) stimulated

TTAP Method steps	Learning style(s) used	Brain region(s) stimulated
Step 1: Conversation	Linguistic, interpersonal	Broca's area
Step 2: Music and meditation	Musical, interpersonal	Temporal lobe
Step 3: Drawing and painting	Visual, intrapersonal	Parietal lobe
Step 4: Sculpture	Spatial, kinesthetic	Cerebellum, Motor cortex (gross motor), Temporal lobe
Step 5: Movement and dance	Kinesthetic	Cerebellum, Motor cortex (gross motor), Temporal lobe
Step 6: Personal or group writing experience	Linguistic	Frontal lobe (fine motor), Wernicke's area
Step 7: Food experience	Spatial, kinesthetic	Sensory cortex, Reticular formation
Step 8: Theme event	Visual, kinesthetic interpersonal, intrapersonal	Reticular formation
Step 9: Phototherapy	Visual, intrapersonal	Broca's area
Step 10: Sensory stimulation	Spatial, kinesthetic, musical, linguistic, interpersonal, intrapersonal	All brain regions
Step 11: Drama or theater experience	Spatial, kinesthetic, musical, linguistic, interpersonal, intrapersonal	All brain regions
Step 12: Client feedback, assessment, evaluation	Any level the participant is capable of writing or responding verbally	Frontal lobe, Wernicke's area

lates directly with Alzheimer's: Modern imaging technology has identified which brain regions, and therefore which cognitive and physical functions, are directly affected during the progression of the disease (see Chapters 1 and 3). With respect to the TTAP Method, Table 5.2 shows each step of the process in relation to which brain region is stimulated and which learning styles are used.

Based on an understanding of the geography of the brain and the regions that respond to specific stimulation, the therapist can design and implement activities for individuals with Alzheimer's. For example, the affective system contains the limbic system, which is responsible for emotions such as happiness, joy, fear, sorrow, contentment, and depression. The therapist can implement thematic programming to elicit specific emotions, which is good for the brain. (See the section "Emotions and Brain Stimulation" later in this chapter.) The retrieval of long-term memories, a skill that people with Alzheimer's possess to varying degrees throughout the disease process, is one of the best ways in which this is accomplished. Therefore, creating thematic programming from memories of childhood, holidays, school, vacations, and so forth is not only beneficial from a participatory perspective but is also very healthful for the brain. With respect to the strategic system, whose primary functions are speaking, hearing, reading, using fine motor skills, and planning, the TTAP Method uses graphic organizers structured around a particular theme to encourage participants to share and express their thoughts as a way to exercise this area of the brain directly (see Chapter 3). For example, asking participants to write out their thoughts in a creative poetry class can be used to combine skills controlled by the strategic system. Regarding the recognition system, which identifies associations such as a picture to a word and objects to sounds and patterns, the TTAP Method uses music as a way to stimulate the identification of objects. Another association that can be stimulated through the TTAP Method is that of representing objects using clay, plaster, and papier-mâché.

Research has also defined two types of learning and shown how what a person is learning affects different regions of the brain (Eslinger & Damasio, 1986). Learning was examined in patients with Alzheimer's and in normal controls. The results support the existence of two relatively independent learning systems: *declarative knowledge*, which is knowing, for example, that Boston is the capital of Massachusetts, and *procedural knowledge*, which is knowing how to drive a car. Researchers have identified the specific regions stimulated by these different learning styles (Eslinger & Damasio, 1986). The declarative knowledge system appears to be associated with corticotemporal/limbic structures, and the procedural system likely depends on the corticocerebellar/striatal structures. These findings parallel current research on how specific regions are stimulated and support the proposition that people, specifically those diagnosed with Alzheimer's, can better exercise their brain by participating in both types of learning processes.

The TTAP Method incorporates both declarative and procedural learning. Through each step participants are repeatedly exposed to declarative knowledge by defining what the topic and theme of the conversation and activities are. Simultaneously, individuals learn the "how to" of each creative experience. The TTAP Method includes continuous invitations to recall, which has been proven to enhance neural connections, and consequently to enhance cognitive reserve (Kensinger, Brierley, Medford, Growdon, & Corkin, 2002) (Figure 5.1).

Those working with people with Alzheimer's quickly learn that within a group are individuals with varying needs, capabilities, and intellect. Understanding how and why people learn individually and within a group, and knowing the effects of therapeutic activities on cognitive functioning, are important in the development and implementation of therapeutic interactions for people diagnosed with

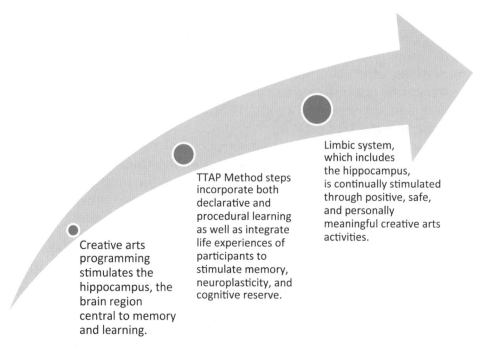

Figure 5.1. How the TTAP Method stimulates cognitive functioning.

Alzheimer's or other dementias. The following sections discuss how emotions and creativity elicited through therapeutic activities can stimulate significant cognitive responses in people with Alzheimer's.

EMOTIONS AND BRAIN STIMULATION

The science and understanding of emotions are difficult to define. Brain imaging and brain stimulation research, however, have demonstrated that emotions and memory are very closely linked (see Chapter 4). You know this from your own experience. Go to a party, meet a bunch of new people. Which faces are you going to remember? The woman who made you laugh or the man who made you feel embarrassed? We remember interactions, both positive and negative, that had an emotional impact. A person is more likely to recall an emotionally arousing event (the death of a loved one, the birth of a child) rather than similar, neutral events (Reisberg & Heuer, 1992). As discussed in Chapter 4, studies indicate that negative emotions (stress, depression, anxiety) have a direct effect in shrinking the hippocampus, the area of the brain that forms complex memories, whereas positive emotions and memories have the opposite effect. The brain responds to positive emotions by releasing estrogen, which plays a crucial role in the stimulation of the hippocampus (Mori et al., 1999). These research findings support the importance of daily opportunities for life review, reminiscence, social interaction, and so forth for people with Alzheimer's to stimulate cognitive functioning and thereby enhance memory (Phelps, 2004). (See Chapter 6 for discussions of life review and reminiscence for people with Alzheimer's.)

Using the TTAP Method, the therapist can structure programming to elicit specific emotions, which is healthful for the brain, in terms of cognitive functioning, memory storage, and recall. Expressing emotions through color, form, shape, and image also releases memories. Using art can enable a person to connect, possibly for the first time, to an emotion or event that has not been thought of for decades.

CREATIVITY AND BRAIN STIMULATION

As discussed in Chapter 3, brain research has shown that continual stimulation of memory, both short and long term, plays an integral role in the wellness of the brain and thus in overall quality of life, including decreased heart rate, increased brain activity in specific pleasure areas of the brain, and an overall sense of well-being. Having a diagnosis of Alzheimer's does not mean that a person cannot share important and relevant experiences and thoughts through a creative outlet. Creativity and the desire for self-expression remain intact throughout the disease process. A growing number of studies indicate that engaging in creative activities, despite the loss of cognitive abilities, can possibly improve cognitive functioning (Alders & Levine Madori, 2010; Hass-Cohen & Carr, 2008; Levine Madori, 2007). Creative expression also enhances interactions between people with Alzheimer's and their family members and caregivers. Actually having something to do has been shown to decrease anxiety and enhance interactions between individuals with Alzheimer's and their caregivers (Truscott, 2004).

Chapter 2 introduced the concept of *flow* and described how an optimal experience of flow contributes to a person's emotional, psychological, social, and physical wellness. The deep concentration and intense involvement that are a part of "being in the flow" stimulate the frontal lobe, specifically the left side (the analytical side, which deals with problem solving), while also stimulating the right frontal lobe (the artistic, creative side) (Levine Madori, 2009). The structure of themed activity and the opportunity to continually revisit themes give the participant a heightened ability to concentrate and focus, thus promoting optimal brain wellness. Immersion in the creative process also fosters a natural loss of self-consciousness, in part because of the positive emotional responses that are elicited through stimulation of the limbic system. The creative process through the TTAP Method has also been documented to enhance psychosocial well-being, self-esteem, and satisfaction (Alders & Levine Madori, 2010; Levine Madori, 2007, 2009). The creative process is the only documented activity that has the ability to distort the sense of time (Csikszentmihalyi, 1997). People who engage in a creative process lose the sense of time and place. Thus disengagement and engagement occur simultaneously. More positive feelings, a state of emotional well-being, and a deep sense of comfort each directly stimulate the brain's neocortex, frontal lobe, occipital lobe, and limbic system.

The creative arts provide a natural balance between level of ability and level of challenge for people with Alzheimer's. The disease itself robs the person of what he or she was able to do before, whereas the creative process allows the person to participate at a level he or she feels comfortable with in the moment. Creative expression not only stimulates cognitive processes but also creates many opportunities for participants to express verbally their experiences of a creative activity, a skill that is under assault throughout the disease process. Encouraging verbal expression through the TTAP Method stimulates both the Broca's and Wernicke's areas of the brain, which are responsible for speech and reading, respectively.

Creativity adds a dimension of vitality and positivity to what at times can be a painful and somewhat tedious experience that people with Alzheimer's and their family members and caregivers face. The simple act of interaction is often difficult and strained. Creative opportunities, such as those offered by the TTAP Method, which are intrinsically rewarding, create opportunities for life review and engage people with Alzheimer's creatively at any level, can directly contribute to overall quality of life at any stage of the disease process.

CONCLUSION

The research and theories of Bloom and Gardner demonstrate how the brain functions and how it stores and processes information. In addition, research has shown that outward stimulations can enhance the physiological and biological aspects of the brain. The cells deep within the hippocampus multiply from visual, verbal, kinesthetic, and tactile stimulation. The brain's ability to regenerate cells offers a new understanding of how to slow the progression of Alzheimer's. If the brain receives continual stimulation through activities that range from crossword puzzles to chess to painting to dance to music to reading, then cell growth is fostered, thereby keeping the brain connections alive, flowing, and multiplying.

The TTAP Method has a dual focus through the creative process: (1) to include all seven learning styles and (2) to stimulate simultaneously all areas of the brain. Furthermore, by incorporating and stimulating each of the three brain systems—affective, strategic, and recognition—the TTAP Method provides participants with continual cognitive stimulation, thereby enhancing learning and recall. Evidence of this process was shown in a 2008 Harvard University study. The ability of older adults to recall detailed memories increased when they were exposed repeatedly to imaginary scenarios (Addis, Wong & Schacter, 2008). According to the researchers, episodic memory, which represents our personal memories of past experiences, "allows individuals to project themselves both backward and forward in subjective time." (Addis, Wong & Schacter, 2008, p. 35) Therefore, in order to create imagined future events, a person must be able to remember the details of previously experienced ones, extract various details, and then put them together to create an imaginary event. This artistic imagery process creates a strong social network that has been noted to increase verbal interactions (Fiore, Becker & Coppel, 1983). These verbal interactions can regulate functions in the cerebral cortex that may be out of reach due to inhibited neural responses attributed to Alzheimer's.

Additionally, the TTAP Method systematically stimulates the hippocampus region, thus slowing the deterioration of memory functioning. The stimulation of memory has been shown to not only delay the progression of Alzheimer's but also to improve some cognitive functioning for a longer period of time (Sabat, 2006). Other studies have suggested that the TTAP Method's structure, which increases verbalization because the group participants are continually encouraged to share and express thoughts that hold significant meaning to them, creates a rewarding emotional experience that may access and stimulate brain cells on a deeper emotional level. For example, in her work with Hispanic older adults diagnosed with Alzheimer's, Alders found the same results after 12 weeks of art therapy sessions using the TTAP Method: "Group participants shared very deep, personal experiences, that went beyond the normal group cohesiveness during the 12 weeks" (Alders, 2009). Participants engaging in the TTAP Method naturally express and represent themselves by sharing past memories, a process that allows them to project themselves both backward and forward in subjective time, continually supporting positive memories and building emotional bonds in the face of Alzheimer's.

The TTAP Method for People with Moderate Alzheimer's: Bergen Regional Medical Center

In 2009, recreation therapists at a skilled nursing facility at the Bergen Regional Medical Center in New Jersey developed session protocols based on the TTAP Method for a 7-week intervention focused on the retention and strengthening of skills and abilities of people diagnosed with moderate to severe Alzheimer's. The study was conducted by fourth-year therapeutic recreation students from St. Thomas Aquinas College in New York. Eight residents participated in the study.

Through verbal responses to questionnaires, the participants gave positive feedback on how engaged they felt during each creative session. Students collected data from the questionnaires and from one open-ended statement from each participant after each session. Each session was found to increase participants' self-esteem and to stimulate multiple aspects of cognitive functioning. The session protocols incorporated the following steps of the TTAP Method: (1) conversation; (2) music and meditation; (3) drawing; (4) sculpture; (5) movement or dance; (6) words, poetry, and stories; and (7) food. Table 5.3 identifies the TTAP Method steps used in each of the seven sessions, the creative arts activity for each step, the learning style each step incorporated, and the brain regions that each step stimulated.

The study was designed to give participants the opportunity to have a voice during each session and to gain insight into their experiences of each activity. The study outcomes demonstrated that, although the participants had significant cognitive impairment, they were able to express positive responses to their experiences of each session. Responses to the open-ended questions showed interesting and powerful evidence of how participants could still engage, describe, and differentiate the sessions from their normal daily activities. As an indication of focused mental stimulation, each person expressed joy in participating in the activities, specifically those diagnosed with moderate Alzheimer's. The sessions revealed the participants' remaining

Table 5.3. Bergen Regional Medical Center study sessions by TTAP Method steps used, learning styles incorporated, and brain regions stimulated

Session	TTAP Method steps	Activity	Learning style	Brain region stimulated
1 (drawing)	2,1,3	(step 2) Therapist plays soft music and takes residents through a body relaxation and guided imagery (theme of which correlates to the activity). (step 1) Therapist discusses guided imagery and meditation with residents, asking questions such as "What did you see?" "Who were you with?" "How did you feel?" (step 3) Residents are given large sheets of paper and different colored markers and are asked to draw a picture. Residents are told they can draw anything they want and that there are no rules or limits to what they can draw.	(step 2) musical/intrapersonal (step 1) linguistic/interpersonal (step 3) visual/intrapersonal	(step 2) Temporal lobe (step 1) Broca's area (step 3) Parietal lobe
2 (sculpture)	2,1,4	(step 2) See description for Session 1. (step 1) See description for Session 1. (step 4) Residents are given a small wooden box and paints and are asked to decorate the box any way they want. They are told that they can put items that they have memories of in the box, or anything else they choose.	(step 2) musical/intrapersonal (step 1) linguistic/interpersonal (step 4) spatial/kinesthetic	(step 2) Temporal lobe (step 1) Broca's area (step 4) Cerebellum, Motor cortex, Temporal lobe
3 (drawing)	2,1,3	(step 2) See description for Session 1. (step 1) See description for Session 1. (step 3) Residents are given a large sheet of paper and small colored shapes. They make a collage out of the shapes by gluing them onto the paper in whatever pattern they choose.	(step 2) musical/intrapersonal (step 1) linguistic/interpersonal (step 3) visual/intrapersonal	(step 2) Temporal lobe (step 1) Broca's area (step 3) Parietal lobe

		Description	Multiple Intelligences	Brain Areas
4 (painting)	2.1.3	(step 2) See description for Session 1. (step 1) See description for Session 1. (step 3) A mask is given to each resident. They use paint to decorate the mask to their liking. Afterward, they are asked to make up a story about their mask and share the story with the group.	(step 2) musical/intrapersonal (step 1) linguistic/interpersonal (step 3) visual/intrapersonal	(step 2) Temporal lobe (step 1) Broca's area (step 3) Parietal lobe
5 (sculpture)	2.1.4	(step 2) See description for Session 1. (step 1) See description for Session 1. (step 4) Residents are given modeling clay and are guided in creating a pumpkin. They then paint the pumpkin to their liking.	(step 2) musical/intrapersonal (step 1) linguistic/interpersonal (step 4) spatial/kinesthetic	(step 2) Temporal lobe (step 1) Broca's area (step 4) Cerebellum, Motor cortex, Temporal lobe
6 (dance)	2.1.5	(step 2) See description for Session 1. (step 1) See description for Session 1. (step 5) Therapist plays music that the residents would remember from their past. Residents are encouraged to get up and dance, if they are able, or to simply move their arms and legs in their seats.	(step 2) musical/intrapersonal (step 1) linguistic/interpersonal (step 5) kinesthetic	(step 2) Temporal lobe (step 1) Broca's area (step 5) Cerebellum, Motor cortex (gross motor), Temporal lobe
7 (words/ poetry)	2.1.6	(step 2) See description for Session 1. (step 1) See description for Session 1. (step 6) Therapist asks residents to come up with a single theme, as well as words that remind them of that theme. Residents then create a story/poem using the words that remind them of the theme.	(step 2) musical/intrapersonal (step 1) linguistic/interpersonal (step 6) linguistic	(step 2) Temporal lobe (step 1) Broca's area (step 6) Frontal lobe (fine motor), Wernicke's area
8 (food)	2.1.7	(step 2) See description for Session 1. (step 1) See description for Session 1. (step 7) Residents get to choose from a variety of food and drinks to celebrate their well-being and the completion of the program sessions!	(step 2) musical/intrapersonal (step 1) linguistic/interpersonal (step 7) spatial/kinesthetic	(step 2) Temporal lobe (step 1) Broca's area (step 7) Sensory cortex, Reticular formation

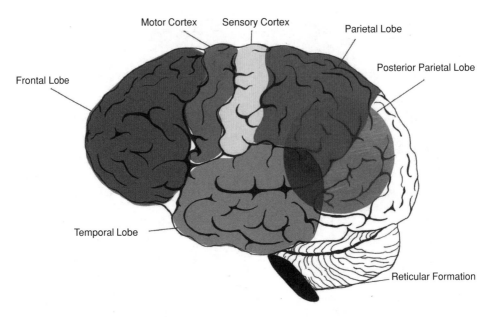

Figure 5.2.   Illustration of brain regions stimulated as part of a theme event (step 8). (Illustration by Lea Madori.)

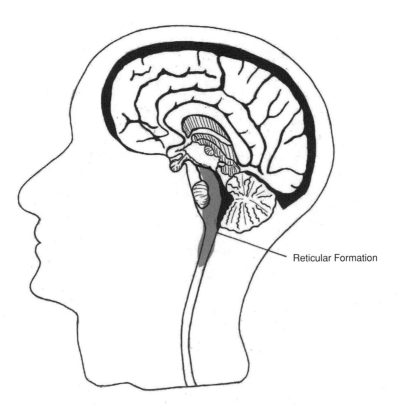

Figure 5.3.   Illustration of brain regions stimulated as part of a sensory stimulation program (step 10). (Illustration by Lea Madori.)

strengths and abilities through self-expression and creativity as well as their desire to engage in the activities rather than to withdraw. Their full attendance at every session throughout the 7 weeks was a testament to their commitment and to the positive, rewarding feelings that resulted.

Results

Participants shared through the verbal questionnaires that each session met their emotional and social needs, with a mean rating of 4.9 out of 5. In addition, students observed the residents gradually interacting more and becoming more verbally active with each other after each session. Not only was there 100% attendance, but also staff noted that residents waited at the elevator to be taken to the session. Participants expressed that they felt "more alive each week" and that they had "a purpose in coming to this program." As part of a recorded interview after the fourth session, some participants stated that they felt they were "doing mental work" and that "this session felt like my brain was being worked out." Other recorded comments included the following: "I felt free during this group"; "I feel very happy"; "I was able to really create something"; "I was able to do what I wanted"; "Someone saved me a lot of trouble"; "I would like to be more active but I am not right now"; "I am becoming more active coming to this program"; "I am always active."

The TTAP Method sessions were found to increase the residents' overall quality of life and personal satisfaction by allowing their voices to be heard. Also, from the first to the last session, resident verbalizations and use of language measurably increased. By stimulating specific brain regions as well as by incorporating each of the seven styles of learning, each session created opportunities for cognitive stimulation.

CHAPTER 6

Aging and Human Developmental Theories

Understanding and Meeting the Needs of Older Adults, Including Those with Dementia

Professional and family caregivers understand more and more the importance of person-centered care approaches for people with Alzheimer's and other dementias. The TTAP Method incorporates several different aging, developmental, and psychological perspectives that support the idea of person-centered care. If a person has an interest, there is intrinsic motivation, and this intrinsic motivation drives the individual into action. The TTAP Method provides direction and assists art and recreation therapists in finding "windows" into the past interests and experiences of those with dementia. These windows guide the therapist in further exploring a person's past interests and experiences by incorporating them into programming now and in the future.

This chapter will review several aging, developmental, and psychological theories and how each informs the TTAP Method in meeting the needs of those with Alzheimer's disease and other forms of dementia. Two distinct areas comprise the theoretical underpinnings for the TTAP Method: (1) theories on aging, which stress the importance of engaging in activities throughout the life span, and (2) theories on psychological development. Developmental theory and life-span theory explain why humans do what they do. These theories are also the theoretical bases from which therapeutic recreation has grown. Having an understanding of the theoretical concepts and foundations of the TTAP Method enables the therapist to create a programming structure that enhances an individual's perceived freedom through personal choice, intrinsic motivation through self-determination, and self-efficacy. The chapter concludes with a discussion of the evolution of the TTAP Method as a taxonomy, or classification, of learning and cognitive stimulation for people with Alzheimer's disease and other dementias.

DEVELOPMENTAL THEORY

Erik Erikson (1963) provided a basis for understanding the significance of change at different times throughout the life span. He suggested that development of self is a continuous process defined by critical periods during which aspects of a person's identity and personality emerge and change. Erikson classified developmental theory into eight psychological stages or tasks of life (Erikson, Erikson, & Kivnick, 1986):

1. Infancy: Trust versus mistrust

2. Childhood: Autonomy versus shame

3. Play age: Initiative versus guilt

4. School age: Industry versus inferiority

5. Adolescence: Identity versus confusion

6. Young adulthood: Intimacy versus isolation

7. Adulthood: Generativity versus self-absorption

8. Old age: Ego integrity versus despair

In 1983, as Erikson himself was reaching old age, he added the eighth psychological stage to his original seven. He described old age as the time during which a person reflects back on his or her life as it has been lived, with the goal of achieving *ego integrity*. By this he meant that if an individual lives long enough and resolves all the earlier tasks of adulthood—such as developing a viable identity and a close and satisfying intimacy and passing on genes and values through generations—the last remaining task that is essential for a person's full development as a human being consists of bringing together a meaningful story about his or her past and present and reconciling with the approaching end of life. If in the later years one looks back with puzzlement and regret, unable to accept the choices made and wishing for another chance, then despair is likely to ensue. But if a person is able to accept his or her unique life, all that has been experienced and all that can be relived through memory, then he or she can achieve a state of ego integrity, or self-acceptance.

Self-growth is an essential element of each of Erikson's psychological stages. Older adults can experience self-growth through leisure and recreational pursuits that allow opportunities for significant meaning to be drawn from past experiences and used in the process of achieving ego integrity. Contrary to common belief, this process is also possible for people with Alzheimer's and other forms of dementia, whose remaining skills and abilities throughout the disease process include the ability to tap into long-term memories, which can be further enhanced through structured art and recreation programming.

Erikson (1963) specifically addressed physical deterioration in aging but theorized that ego integrity can be mastered through cognitive processes, regardless of physical status. For people to approach or experience integrity, they must be actively involved in society, community, or personal pursuits and interests that continually stimulate them. He wrote that "elders who live their lives to the fullest, participating in activities on a day-to-day basis, uncertain of or unwilling to count on the future . . . continue to behave in a fashion that takes a future for granted" (p. 58). This understanding of the human experience in the last stage of life speaks directly to the importance of being engaged in activities on a daily basis.

Erikson's concept (1963) of ego integrity includes an implied wellness of the ego that consists of a balance between emotional, social, and physical states of mind. This concept of wellness (the culmination of a sense of acceptance of oneself and a feeling of fulfillment) is reflected in three areas. First, personal fulfillment is found in the actions of the individual, in freedom of choice, and in direct action related to preferences. Second, the ability to attain wellness resides in the roles through which a person lives and interacts with others. Third, wellness can be achieved through one's ability to live (by direct action in personal pursuits) with an overall feeling of wellness. These concepts form the foundation and philosophy of therapeutic recreation for individuals with Alzheimer's and other dementias. (Chapter 2 discusses how these wellness concepts are interrelated and woven into the TTAP Method.)

Paralleling Erikson's work, Butler (1963) incorporated the concept of ego integrity in characterizing the inner process that an aging adult experiences. Butler defined ego integrity as a universal process in older people that is stimulated by aging: "Important memories and feelings are revived in order to resolve current or past conflicts" (p. 66). Both Butler and Erikson proposed that the tendency of older adults to review their past has a positive psychological, emotional, and cognitive impact on the developmental process of ego integrity and enhances feelings of well-being.

Erikson (1963) stated that *activities* are fundamental channels through which the individual integrates and processes life experiences and thereby achieves self-acceptance and feelings of fulfillment. Erikson and colleagues (1986) further elaborated that positive development in the last stage of life must be promoted by the individual or by the community in which the person resides: "Continued growth and development throughout old age is reinforced by either personal contributions by the individual toward their family, friends, and society or by acquiring new skills and attitudes that allow feelings of personal contribution" (p. 270). Activities that are recreational, educational, or therapeutic are significant to human growth and development and promote emotional, social, cognitive, and physical well-being at any age; they are, however, even more significant in old age (Butler, 1963; Erikson, 1963; Erikson et al., 1986).

LIFE-SPAN THEORY

Developed by Paul Baltes, a developmental psychologist, life-span theory expands on developmental theory by viewing human development in relation to the following principles:

Lifelong: People have the potential for development throughout their life span.

Multidimensional: Development crosses multiple dimensions, including social, emotional, cognitive, and biological.

Multidirectional: Human development is not always forward; people experience gains and losses at all ages.

Multidisciplinary: Development must be considered in the context of many disciplines, including medical, psychological, and behavioral.

Plastic: People have the ability to change and adapt, thus producing plasticity or variability in their behavior and development.

Contextual: Development is influenced by the context of a person's environment (family, physical environment, educational influences, cultural and societal norms) and by historical time and place (Butterworth, 1994).

Baltes et al. (1980) distinguished three types of influences on the individual: (1) normative (age grade), (2) normative historical (evolutionary), and (3) nonnormative. All three "mediate through the developing individual, act and interact to produce life-span development" (p. 75). Baltes defines *normative* influence as a person's actual age; *normative historical* as a person's past or history (e.g., job, interests, and social, community, or spiritual pursuits); and *nonnormative* as the state that one is in as a result of unforeseen physical, psychological, or emotional disturbances. Consider the case of Jose, who was moved into a skilled nursing facility (SNF) after being diagnosed with moderate Alzheimer's. His normative age at the time he moved was 79. Before retiring and then having the accident that led to his move to the SNF, Jose had served for many years as a maintenance man for a local community college. He had enjoyed the labor and rewards of servicing the needs of the buildings, the instructors, and the students. He took pride in maintaining the appearance and functioning of these public facilities and he enjoyed the social interactions with the various members of the college community. The nonnormative state for Jose is that at roughly 80 years old he finds himself suddenly among old people who do not look at one another, do not speak to one another, and slowly turn inward, acting as old as someone 100 years old and ready to die. Jose is still a vital and virile man. He helps push others in wheelchairs and assists with moving furniture, activities that reflect the historical nature of life-span theory, in their correlation between Jose's interests while he is living at the SNF and his interests before moving to the facility. Also, a person's past activity levels can predict future activity levels (Scarmeas et al., 2001). Therefore, including history-graded (evolutionary) influences (defined as biological and environmental elements) clarifies an individual's development through his or her changing physical body coupled with a changing environment or world.

Voelkl and Mathieu (1995) and Voelkl and colleagues (1996) used life-span theory as a theoretical framework to analyze the activity level of residents of SNFs. Residents were asked to identify in interviews and on an activity checklist the leisure activities in which they participated before and after moving to the SNF. Voelkl and Mathieu's research documented a strong statistical correlation between high levels of activity participation before entering an SNF and high levels of activity levels after moving to the SNF and demonstrated consistency in activity participation throughout the life span. Their findings support life-span theory (Baltes et al., 1980) with this association between activity level in earlier stages of life and in the last stage of life.

Life-span theory was also the theoretical framework for the Nun Study (Lemonick & Park, 2001; Snowdon, 2001 [described in detail in Chapter 4]), which is the largest, longest (participants' ages ranged from 16 years to death), and most significant research to date linking cognition, education, and recreational activities to life-span development. The behaviors (e.g., art and recreation activities, praying, writing, reading) of 678 nuns were followed by Snowdon from the time the nuns entered the convent at age 16. The study strongly demonstrated the relationship between activity participation and wellness. The nuns who participated more frequently in therapeutic activities were less likely to have dementia-related illness as they grew older.

Life-span development theory, therefore, helps to underscore the important role leisure activities can play in the lives of all older adults, including residents in long-term care communities, and moreover the importance of activities that allow individuals to express and experience past interests. These concepts closely parallel the goals of the TTAP Method to offer multiple opportunities for people with Alzheimer's and other dementias to move from current situations (the present) into the past or the future through structured thematic programming activities.

RECREATION

In addition to being grounded by developmental and life-span theories, the TTAP Method grows out of the principles and practices of therapeutic recreation. The field of therapeutic recreation applies a humanistic approach to the conceptual frameworks of developmental and life-span theories. An understanding of what therapeutic recreation encompasses must begin with an understanding of what is meant by *recreation*. Kraus (1978) defined recreational activities or experiences as those that usually are chosen voluntarily by the participant either because of the pleasure or creative enrichment that is derived from them or because of a perception that personal or social value will be gained. The recreation experience, although often within a group environment, is individual and unique.

The use of recreational activities as a therapeutic adjunct to care was first introduced in facilities for people with mental disabilities in the mid-1900s. Avedon (1974) explained the development of therapeutic recreation and proposed the concept of therapeutic recreation service to prevent dysfunctions that result from a lack of recreation opportunities among special groups and to treat illness and disability.

Austin (2001) explained that "[therapeutic recreation] recognizes the importance of having the ability to be self-directed by taking action. The freedom to make independent choices based on personal preferences is essential to develop themselves through the involvement or action of therapeutic activities across the life span" (pp. 33, 149). One essential concept in therapeutic recreation is the ability of individuals to progress across a continuum of wellness when the activities are therapeutic or educational in nature or pursued on the basis of personal preference. This continuum of wellness was described by Peterson and Gunn (1984) within the framework of health and illness: An individual, throughout the life span, can pass from wellness to illness and back again.

According to the National Therapeutic Recreation Society, which was established in 1982, the purpose of therapeutic recreation is to facilitate the development, maintenance, and expression of an appropriate leisure lifestyle for individuals with physical, cognitive, emotional, and/or social limitations. Research on therapeutic recreation as part of a care plan has been conducted since the early 1980s, and it has been shown to have a significant and positive effect on well elderly individuals and residents in assisted living centers.

Since the early 1990s, researchers have additionally proven that therapeutic recreation has a positive effect on individuals diagnosed with varying stages of Alzheimer's disease, producing positive outcomes on cognition, socialization, and physical and emotional well-being in residents of SNFs. Specific studies have focused on cognitive functioning (Buettner, Kernan, & Carroll, 1990), psychosocial well-being (Voelkl & Mathieu, 1995), and physical functioning (Cohen-Mansfield, Werner, & Rosenthal, 1992).

Research by Levine Madori (2004) with individuals who spent one full year in an SNF and were diagnosed with only mild or moderate Alzheimer's disease revealed both positive and significant correlations between cognition and psychosocial well-being as time involved in programming and frequency of participation in varying therapeutic recreation activities increased. Therapeutic recreation also has been shown to have a positive psychological effect on individuals with severe Alzheimer's disease (Dunn & Wilhite, 1997; Weiss & Kronberg, 1986).

According to developmental and life-span theories, individuals who have Alzheimer's disease and face the threat of loss of self as well as death still can attain ego integrity. Through active participation in therapeutic activities, these individuals can have positive experiences that promote emotional well-being, enhance physical capabilities, and improve overall psychosocial well-being. Concepts of therapeutic recreation that are derived from developmental and life-span theories include providing continual promotion of self-driven choices, intrinsic motivation, optimal experiences, self-actualization through freedom of self-expression, and facilitation in achieving the fullest possible growth and overall development (Austin, 2001), all of which have the potential for actualization in people with dementia and all of which are incorporated into TTAP Method programming.

THE CONTINUUM OF PSYCHOLOGICAL DOMAINS

To discuss therapeutic art and recreation programming for persons with dementia, it is important first to understand the aging individual in a specific point in time along the spectrum of the life span. Many researchers in the field of developmental psychology have written about and documented five domains that directly make up human existence: cognitive, emotional, physical, spiritual, and social. These domains are the basic components on which therapeutic interventions can be based when one is developing individual and group programs for persons with dementia. Therapists have always discussed the fundamental principles

Table 6.1. The Continuum of Psychological Domains

Value	Well elderly	Assisted living	Skilled Nursing	Dementia	Hospice Care
5 (high)	Social	Emotional	Cognitive	Physical	Spiritual
4	Emotional	Cognitive	Physical	Cognitive	Cognitive
3	Cognitive	Physical	Social	Emotional	Emotional
2	Physical	Social	Emotional	Social	Social
1 (low)	Spiritual	Spiritual	Spiritual	Spiritual	Physical

that each psychological domain encapsulates; however, the concept of using these domains together or separately as significant compositional structures in developing individual programming needs, goals, and objectives for persons with dementia has not been addressed in art or recreation therapy. The TTAP Method addresses the clients' specific needs in the five domains by programming directly to those needs. Constructing and designing thematic programming for the Alzheimer's population must begin with assessing which domain(s) should be highlighted for this cohort at each stage of the disease progression.

I developed the Continuum of Psychological Domains (Table 6.1) to express the changing importance of each domain at each stage in the aging process: well aging in the community, aging in assisted living, aging in skilled nursing, and aging with cognitive disabilities. As one moves from independence to dependence, so, too, does the importance of each domain shift from social to emotional to cognitive to physical to spiritual. Although certain psychological domains take preeminence at each stage, the continuum also reveals the necessity of assessing the individual for all domains so the therapist can serve each person to the best of his or her abilities. The person with Alzheimer's disease continues to possess strengths and abilities that therapeutic interventions can tap into to help meet his or her social, emotional, cognitive, physical, and spiritual needs.

I derived the concept of the Continuum of Psychological Domains from Engel's Biopsychosocial Model, which considers a disease or physical condition not only as manifesting in terms of pathophysiology but also simultaneously affecting many levels of functioning, from cellular to organ to person to family to society (Engel, 1977). Alzheimer's disease and other dementias are prime examples of this phenomenon. The biopsychosocial model was the first to provide a broader understanding of the disease process as encompassing multiple levels of functioning, including the therapist–client or doctor–patient relationship. Engel's model emphasizes that change in one area of an individual's life will affect other areas, which is certainly the case with the progression of Alzheimer's.

Returning to the CCDERS Approach™ introduced in Chapter 2, the TTAP Method incorporates and promotes the following six common strengths and abilities that an individual with Alzheimer's possesses throughout the disease process:

Communicate with others

Connect with others

Differentiate likes and dislikes

Express feelings and emotions

Recall long-term memories

Self-express pleasurable emotions and receiving joy

Successful thematic programming for individuals with dementia emphasizes and draws from the cognitive abilities that the individual still has left. It is extremely important to focus on what the individual can still do to lessen his or her frustration or to even prevent it from occurring. Dementia takes away so very much of a person's ability to function that each person must be assessed individually to find remaining strengths.

The Continuum of Psychological Domains can be used by the therapist in assessing the specific needs of the individual and then designing programming specifically for each domain. As the Continuum illustrates, in the process of normal aging, social interaction directly affects emotional outcomes, and through emotional gratification, we are moved toward cognitive and physical stimulation. This is the basic principle for understanding and incorporating thematic programming into therapeutic domains. Each individual is unique and different; the Continuum of Psychological Domains is designed to be a "jumping off" or starting point from which the therapist can better assess and design therapeutic interventions to focus on the remaining strengths of those with dementia.

The Continuum of Psychological Domains for the Individual with Dementia

As emphasized throughout this book, research has shown that continual and challenging cognitive stimulation is the key to slowing the progression of neurodegeneration for people with Alzheimer's and other dementias. With this in mind, it makes sense to begin TTAP Method programming in the physical domain where the individual still feels capable of following simple directions and deriving great pleasure from socializing within a group, as illustrated below:

Physical → Cognitive → Emotional → Social → Spiritual

Moving into cognitive thematic programming brings in personal interests and topics that the residents have had their entire lives. Leading the participants through the TTAP Method thus ensures a rich emotionally and socially stimulating process. Spiritually, residents continue to reach out to the philosophies and religious beliefs that they have known their entire lives.

TTAP Method programming incorporates each psychological domain as follows:

Physical component: Participants actually "do," using fine and gross motor coordination.

Cognitive component: Participants grow to understand and know themselves better by socializing and conversing with others in the group in a safe, supportive group dynamic. Each session stimulates specific regions of the brain through specific actions and thereby enhances cognitive functioning.

Emotional component: Participants continually share feelings and past experiences with others in the group setting. Each individual draws from his or her emotional self in doing so. Research has shown that emotional stimulation directly and effectively stimulates neurodevelopmental growth on a cellular level (brain plasticity) (see Chapter 4).

Social component: Those diagnosed with Alzheimer's begin to regress and find themselves isolated and lacking social interactions. Through the TTAP Method participants are integrated into a group setting by continually giving support to others and receiving support from other group members. Individuals reclaim the ability to learn about and respond to others. Socialization is paramount in slowing cognitive deterioration; the less we socialize the faster we decline cognitively.

Spiritual component: Thematic programming can be used to stimulate participants' recall and sharing of long-term memories and experiences related to spirituality. Additionally, participants recognize their own spirituality in the stories and interactions with others.

As discussed in Chapter 4, researchers have correlated external stimulation with enhanced cognitive functioning and are developing an evolving understanding of the brain's functioning and its ability to regrow cells. Outward stimulation, including through creative arts experiences, can cause cells in different regions of the brain to rejuvenate and regrow. These breakthroughs could dramatically affect the understanding of the importance of therapeutic activities throughout the life span as they relate to and directly affect *brain wellness* (Diamond, 2000). The TTAP Method follows the concept of "use it or lose it," stimulating all aspects of brain functioning while also addressing the needs of the client across the psychological domains.

LIFE REVIEW AND PEOPLE WITH ALZHEIMER'S DISEASE

Returning to Erikson's stages of human development, an important element in achieving ego integrity is *cognitive life review*, a significant mental process by which a person reviews and synthesizes his or her entire life by engaging in stimulating activities (Erikson et al., 1986). Often, therapists facilitate a reminiscence group without really understanding the significance of revisiting life experiences as part of a group. Engagement in activities is as crucial to overall well-being as reminiscence is to a person's psychological well-being.

Numerous studies have shown the usefulness of structured life review in caring for people with Alzheimer's, primarily within the fields of nursing, psychology, and gerontology. Because of similarities in the nature of programs, the term *life review* is often used interchangeably with *reminiscence*, as in *integrative reminiscence*, *guided reminiscence*, and *therapeutic reminiscence* (Mastel-Smith et al., 2006; Wong & Watt, 1991). However, life review differs from simple reminiscence in that it must be structured and comprehensive. Life review also involves an evaluative process that is characterized by the systematic analysis of memories, past conflicts, or unresolved issues. Although reminiscence has therapeutic value, it is not evaluative or episodic, nor sequential, probative, or exhaustive.

Structured life review is most effective when used early in the disease process, when a person is able to attend to the structure more easily and can recall more memories. In the early stages, an individual also has more cognitive function, which is necessary for analyzing memories and resolving past conflicts or issues. Although the life review process is most effective at the beginning of the disease, it is also effective throughout the disease progression. It is possible to conduct a life review with a person in more advanced stages as long as he or she is still able to communicate (Haight, 2007).

Beyond helping those with Alzheimer's achieve ego integrity (an accepted life), encouraging them to recall past memories and experiences in a structured, more orderly fashion helps them to retain more orderly thinking, a skill that declines as the disease progresses. Although it is not one of the goals of a structured life review, orderly thinking may result in improved scores on the Mini-Mental State Exam and in greater self-confidence for someone with Alzheimer's. Changing the way a person with Alzheimer's processes thought (e.g., through an ordered structure) is still possible (Haight, 2007).

Tabourne (1991) developed the Life Review Program (LRP) as a therapeutic recreation intervention to mitigate some of the emotional and psychological problems associated with Alzheimer's. The LRP was shown to successfully reduce disorientation, depression, and poor self-esteem in non-Hispanic white older adults with the disease (Tabourne, 1995), and to increase the psychological well-being of non-Hispanic African-American older adults (McKenzie, 2004). Although the LRP was initially used to study non-Hispanic white older adults, the life review process itself has been shown to enhance emotional well-being and decrease emotional distress in different cultural populations (McKenzie, 1996).

In 2008, Tabourne and colleagues used LRP with a group of 17 Korean older adults diagnosed with Alzheimer's who were still able to follow instructions, participate in activities, and respond with understanding to questions (Lee, Tabourne, & Yoon, 2008). Using patient self-appraisals on functioning, in-depth interviews were conducted to obtain qualitative data and to give each patient a voice. What the participants shared revealed five themes that illustrate how significant life review is for people diagnosed with Alzheimer's:

Theme 1: LRP helped participants go back to their pasts. One person stated, "I could not say anything about my past. . . . I never considered my life to be serious, but this program gave me the opportunity to reconsider about my life, and it was a good time!"

Theme 2: LRP helped participants find meaning in their lives. The participants all shared that it seemed as though they had forgotten about their pasts in that they were not directed to think about their pasts. LRP helped to structure their attention toward the past.

Theme 3: LRP helped participants to reflect on their identities through their accomplishments throughout their lives. All participants shared the common feeling that LRP helped them to think about who they were in terms of what they had accomplished throughout their lives. Discussing the value of their occupational pursuits and the jobs they held was considered a very positive experience. Participants were able to reflect on and define who they were in terms of their accomplishments.

Theme 4: LRP helped participants evaluate their lives with regard to economic success and family success. Participants expressed positive regard toward what they had attained throughout their lives both in economic terms and in the success of the structure and development of their families.

Theme 5: LRP helped to decrease emotional distress for participants. Participants all felt that the LRP offered relief from the stresses of their daily lives. The ability to revisit the past gave them all deep feelings of happiness and joy.

Despite common perceptions about the limitations of a person's ability to be self-reflective in the face of cognitive decline, these themes reveal that LRP held great value for the Alzheimer's study group and that those with the disease can and want to reflect back on their lives and to have a forum in which to be heard.

Life review also has been shown to positively affect mood and well-being (Bohlmeijer, Smit, & Cuijpers, 2003; Haight & Burnside, 1993; Haight et al., 2003; Tabourne, 1991, 1995). A study of institutionalized adults with moderate dementia found that life review promoted memory, enhanced perceived social values of self, decreased disorientation, reduced fear and anxiety, and improved self-esteem and social interaction (Tabourne, 1995). Other studies have demonstrated that structured life review assists in regaining and maintaining a cohesive sense of self, so that people can carry out psychological and social tasks and revise life structures in the context of the illness experience (Bohlmeijer et al., 2005; Haight, 1995). Reminiscence and life review as a therapeutic approach are also useful interventions in treating depression in older adults with dementia (Cappeliez, O'Rourke, & Chaudhury, 2005).

The TTAP Method offers therapists, caregivers, and health care providers simple yet powerful ways in which to use an object or a theme in a progressive way to create multiple, structured opportunities for life review (Levine Madori, 2007, 2009a,b,c). As illustrated in Figure 6.1, the TTAP Method uses two distinct psychological approaches for activating personal memories in people at any stage of Alzheimer's: through objects or through the events related to themes throughout the life span. For example, an object such as a music box that a person enjoys listening to can be used to discuss where the music box came from, who gave it to the person and for what occasion, or why the sounds from the music box are so pleasing. This type of therapeutic

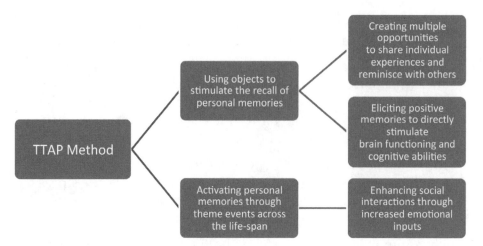

Figure 6.1. The TTAP Method enhances opportunities for life review during programming.

interaction engages the individual by stimulating conversation, memory, and positive life review. (See Chapter 2 for further discussion of the use of the TTAP Method in developing activities that promote life review, including with respect to the CCDERS™ Approach. See Chapter 3 for suggestions of creative arts activities based on phototherapy [step 9 of the TTAP Method].)

Developmental theory and cognitive life review address the significance of activities in later life. Life-span theory goes further to explain that personal pursuits in society and communities foster an emotional, social, physical, and cognitive balance. Through these experiences, a person develops a sense of self-acceptance, which fosters ego integrity. These theories also link improved cognitive functioning to activity participation. Therapeutic recreation using the TTAP Method enables participants to continue to grow and develop, even in the last stage of life and even in the face of Alzheimer's. Life expectancy has increased dramatically in modern time, to the point that the last stage of human life now lasts longer than any other developmental stage. It is critical to realize that the activities in which older adults engage are fundamental to overall, long-term well-being.

The TTAP Method incorporates developmental, life-span, and life review theories on many levels. For example, in step 1 (group conversation), participants engage in structured communication based on a theme or an object that helps each person to focus on the past and recall positive life memories. In step 2 (music and meditation), participants are taken through a guided imagery to a safe, pleasant place in which to experience a favorite piece of music or a special place that he or she enjoyed visiting as a child or young adult. In step 5 (movement and dance), the person is brought back to and grounded in his or her body through movement, dance, and music. Step 6 (group writing experience) can be applied as part of a structured life review; participants can share in writing within the group setting a story or event from their past that relates to a theme. Step 8 (theme event) creates multiple opportunities for participants to create and maintain social bonds, which, as discussed earlier, is essential for preventing self-isolation and for improving cognitive functioning.

Having discussed some of the historical theories that underpin the TTAP Method, the remainder of this chapter will review several more contemporary aging and development theories that also contribute to an understanding of how implementation of the TTAP Method will help professional and family caregivers in meeting the unique needs of the fast-growing number of people with Alzheimer's disease and other forms of dementia.

HUMANISTIC PSYCHOLOGY: THE ORIGIN OF PERSON-CENTERED THEORY

Humanistic psychology was developed in the 1950s in reaction to the then widely held belief that all clients should have the same treatment outcome as a result of traditional behavioral and psychoanalytic approaches, which gave very little thought to the fact that individuals have vastly different experiences and personal resources. Drawing on the philosophies of existentialism and phenomenology, humanistic psychology is a subjective, person-centered perspective on human existence that considers the whole person, focusing on individual needs, strengths, and weaknesses (Rowan, 2001). The basic tenets of humanistic psychology include freedom, choice, values, personal responsibility, purpose, spirituality, self-actualization, and individuality.

One of the founders of the humanistic approach to psychology was Carl Rogers, who in 1964 developed *client-centered therapy* (Bugental, 1964). Now more widely called *person-centered therapy*, it is one of the most extensively used models in psychotherapy today. Person-centered therapy involves showing genuineness, empathy, and unconditional positive regard toward a client in order to establish a supportive, nonjudgmental environment in which the individual is encouraged to reach his or her full potential. As simple as it sounds, this therapy was and remains today a powerful and successful therapeutic intervention, designed to assess a person's specific needs and to incorporate those needs in the development of treatment strategies. Rogers characterized the client's capacity for self-direction and understanding of his or her own development in one of his most influential books, *On Becoming a Person* (1961):

> People are essentially trustworthy, that they have a vast potential for understanding themselves and resolving their own problems without direct intervention on the therapist's part, and that they are capable of self-directed growth if they are involved in a specific kind of therapeutic relationship. (p. 61)

The turn of the century has seen a shift in models of Alzheimer's care away from a medical model to a similar person-centered care philosophy in which a positive relationship is established that incorporates the following four key components:

- Valuing people with dementia and those who care for them
- Treating people with dementia as individuals
- Looking at the world from the perspective of people with dementia
- Providing a positive social environment in which people with dementia can experience relative well-being (Brooker, 2004)

This shift has been accompanied by research that has shown that individuals with Alzheimer's need a therapeutic approach that addresses the following (Bossen, Specht, & McKenzie, 2009):

- To be heard (they maintain awareness much longer than previously assumed)
- To be informed (i.e., of the most recent information on and knowledge of Alzheimer's disease)
- To receive emotional and cognitive support
- To promote health (people with Alzheimer's are highly likely to seek and participate in physical activities)
- To maintain cognitive abilities in the face of difficulties with processing information, task breakdown, memory, sequencing, and decision making

People with Alzheimer's need to be *heard, understood,* and, most important, *responded to* throughout the disease process (Bossen, Specht, & McKenzie, 2009). They have an innate desire to be involved and proactive in determining their needs and having a voice in their plan of care to possibly slow the disease process. Stimulating the brain through person-centered activities and allowing the client a voice are, therefore, essential for client advocacy. Person-centered approaches have been shown to reduce anxiety, depression, agitation, aggression, and discomfort throughout all stages of the disease (Koch, 2004; Sloane, Hoeffer, Madeline, McKenzie, et al., 2004). Alzheimer's has a major impact on social interactions and self-concept; group support is essential. Through the TTAP Method individuals with Alzheimer's can participate at whatever level they feel is comfortable and appropriate while rediscovering themselves through others in the group experience (Sterin, 2002).

How the TTAP Method Incorporates Person-Centered Theory

Effective implementation of person-centered care for people with Alzheimer's disease using the TTAP Method requires a shared understanding and commitment on the part of administrative personnel, direct-care providers, residents, and their family members. The importance of family involvement in person-centered care is critical to each resident's overall wellness (see Chapter 1), and long-term care facilities must seek ways to engage families in person-centered care and activities through training, policies, care planning, and documentation. The TTAP Method offers simple program ideas, protocols, and assessments that can be carried out across the facility, thus allowing family members, for example, to communicate with staff and build consensus and shared values regarding how their loved one is responding, what his or her needs and choices are, and which themed sessions are best suited for him or her. (See Chapter 3 for programming suggestions for each step of the TTAP Method.) The TTAP Method honors the unique perspectives, values, and needs of each resident receiving care. Participation stimulates the brain, which in turn stimulates positive emotions and the ability to continue to strive for positive personal interaction. For example, caregivers on all units can converse with a resident who has Alzheimer's in ways that incorporate the individual's past experiences, thus creating a positive communication cycle. Such an approach has the greatest chance of success in promoting person-centered care and the shared values necessary to ensure its successful implementation (Boise & White, 2004).

Conversation is the fundamental element of the TTAP Method (see Chapter 3). It is imperative to check in with residents, to ask what is on their minds, how they are feeling, or what *they* want to discuss today. If you have completed a meditation session with a resident, ask what he or she would like to do next (e.g., write a story about what came to mind during the meditation; paint or draw an image of something seen or recalled). Every decision a person makes enhances self-esteem through shared choices and decision making. This process takes place through each step of the TTAP Method. Staff can work together to purposefully use themes to enhance communication possibilities with residents (see Chapters 2 and 3). Instead of coming into a room solely to dispense medication, for example, a nurse can use the theme of summertime or summer vacations to engage a resident in a conversation about a favorite vacation spot or summer experience. These more person-centered interactions are rich with possibilities.

NEURODEVELOPMENTAL THEORY AND TREATMENT

The growing knowledge of brain plasticity and how certain activities can stimulate specific brain regions have had a profound influence on the care and treatment of individuals with a neurological disorder or cognitive impairment caused by brain trauma or disease. Modern technology has allowed glimpses into the brain and its functioning that have never before been possible, revealing new knowledge about how regions of the brain communicate and how brain cells degenerate or regenerate. Many of the new theories and treatments that have emerged as a result have first been developed through studies with children, whose brains are still developing. Other studies have focused specifically on the capacity of the adult brain to recover from trauma or disease.

One treatment model that has emerged is neuro-developmental treatment (NDT), which is used to enhance the functional abilities of individuals who have acquired a neurological disorder as a result of a brain trauma (Gault, 2008). NDT is based on the philosophy that functional abilities can be improved through assessment, planning, and hands-on therapeutic interventions. NDT reflects a person-centered care philosophy in that the approach is guided by the client's responses during each treatment session. NDT therapists identify an individual's strengths and impairments and address them in relation to a person's functional abilities and limitations. The therapists also work collaboratively with patients, families, caregivers, and other health care professionals to develop individualized comprehensive treatment programs (http://www.ndta.org/).

An outgrowth of NDT is the neurosequential model of therapeutics (NMT) approach. Clinician and researcher Bruce Perry developed the NMT as a framework for working with traumatized and maltreated children and young adults (Perry, 2006). The approach is used to (1) organize a child's history and current functioning to inform the therapeutic process and meet the needs of the child and (2) match specific therapeutic techniques to a child's developmental stage as well as to the brain region(s) and neural networks that are mediating the child's neuropsychiatric problems. Key to the success of applying the approach is the active participation of parents, caregivers, therapists, and other adults in the child's life. (Perry, 2006, 2009; Perry & Hambrick, 2008; http://childtrauma.org/index.php/services/neurosequential-model-of-therapeutics).

The NMT approach has grown out of current research on brain functioning and cognition that supports the ability of the traumatized brain to reorganize itself by developing new neural connections in response to new stimuli, a process called neuroplasticity (see Chapter 4). Perry (2006, 2008) found that changes occurred at the cellular level in the brain and that brain chemistry was altered when children who had sustained a traumatic brain injury engaged in creative arts activities, such as sculpture, photography, and art. These changes, tracked using PET and CAT scan imaging, showed positive and direct effects of art therapy in treating the neurodevelopmental damage to the brain (Perry, 2001, 2006; Perry, Pollard, Blakely, Baker, & Vigilante, 1995). The process of engaging in creative arts activities promoted the development of new neural connections, which in turn allowed the traumatized child to function at a more optimal social, emotional, and cognitive level. Through his research, Perry identified the following six elements that are necessary for the stimulation of neuronal connections in the brain:

- Relational (safe, stable)
- Relevant (geared to the child's developmental stage, not chronological age)
- Repetitive (creating patterns)
- Rewarding (pleasurable)
- Rhythmic (to affect deep within the brainstem)
- Respectful (of the child, family, and culture)

Building on the success of using art therapy as a therapeutic intervention, Hass-Cohen and Carr (2008) found through their research that the process of engaging in art activities requires an integration of higher cortical thinking, such as planning, attention, mindful problem solving, and social and emotional investment. They further asserted that the art process stimulates specific neurotransmitters in the brain that are responsive to visual and novel stimuli. Art therapy may well promote faster cognitive and emotional processing and facilitate learning and recall while stimulating various other brain functions (Gardner, 1982; Hass-Cohen & Carr, 2008; Kramer, 2000; Kaplan, 2000; De Petrillo & Winner, 2005).

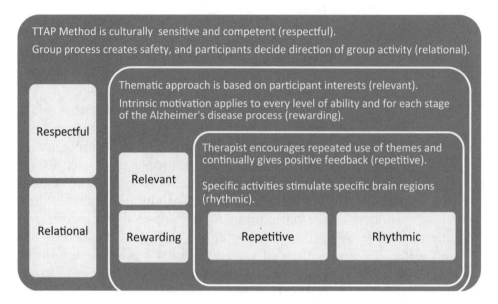

Figure 6.2. The TTAP Method incorporates Perry's six "R's" for stimulating cognitive functioning.

Using the TTAP Method to Enhance Brain Plasticity

As illustrated in Figure 6.2, the TTAP Method incorporates the six elements Perry has shown enhance the brain's ability to create new neural connections, thus optimizing brain wellness and cognitive ability. The continual use of past and present personal interests and life experiences that have accrued across the life span elevates each person's self-expression to a central position in the creative process (respectful). The therapist continually solicits input from the participants through conversation and art experiences, thereby fostering not only participants' free will in choosing to participate but also the extent to which they contribute (relational). Each individual's unique combination of skills, multiple intelligences, and capabilities for self-expression is incorporated (relevant). In the group setting, each step fosters emotional support, stimulating communication, and enriching experiences that provide each person with intrinsic motivation to participate in the creative arts process (rewarding). The therapist encourages within the group the continual use of creativity based on a theme and gives repetitive positive feedback for each step of the process (repetitive). Use of the TTAP Method systematically stimulates the hippocampus region of the brain, as well as other areas, at a deep level by continually engaging a person in visual, auditory, or sensory activities, thus enhancing cognitive functioning (rhythmic).

OBJECT RELATIONS THEORY

Object relations theory emphasizes the role of early childhood experiences in shaping an individual's sense of self. Objects can be real *others* in a person's world (mother and father, siblings, and the like) or *things*, such as transitional objects with which a child forms attachments (stuffed animal, blanket, pet). It is through relationships with these "objects" that the developing child takes in or internalizes parts of others (objects) and slowly builds a sense of self (Klee, 1990). Objects can represent elements of a person's past or present and hold meanings in vastly different ways for everyone. We project our feelings onto objects without being aware of it. Relating to an object can bring to mind thoughts, memories, and feelings that, in the case of a person with Alzheimer's, had been long forgotten.

Object Relations Theory and People with Alzheimer's Disease

Therapeutic interventions based on object relations theory appear helpful in understanding the psyche of a person with Alzheimer's in that an object can trigger an immediate response that can offer a window into the person's soul (Kasl-Godley & Gatz, 2000). An object can be correlated to personal feelings, personal history, and the immediate past. As discussed in Chapters 2 and 3, people with Alzheimer's gradually lose the ability to communicate in relation to person, place, and time. However, an object is not necessarily rooted in any given time or place or in relation to any specific person. For example, a person with Alzheimer's may tie an object to an event or experience that occurred in the 1920s. An example of the usefulness of object relations can be seen in the guided imagery sessions I did with an older man with mild cognitive impairment who was also diagnosed with clinical depression (Box 6.1).

How the TTAP Method Integrates Object Relations Theory

The TTAP Method offers therapists, caregivers, and health care providers simple yet powerful ways in which to use an object to create multiple opportunities for stimulating brain functioning and cognition in people with Alzheimer's. A therapist can incorporate an object into thematic programming by first uncovering aspects of the object in relation to the following three categories (see Figure 6.3):

1. The structure or environment from which the object came (land, sea, air)

Box 6.1.   Using object relations with guided imagery.

This gentleman had recently been admitted into a skilled nursing facility after his wife of 50 years died. He refused to leave his room and spent all his time in bed staring at the ceiling. I visited him daily and tried to converse with him. This became increasingly difficult as he became more and more disconnected and self-isolated. I decided to ask him whether he wanted to do a guided imagery session. He agreed, and so I brought in a CD player to relax him with some music and began his first experience with guided imagery.

Before proceeding, I explained what I would do and told him that he just had to relax and follow my voice. I did the standard garden imagery (see Chapter 3) and ended in a garden. After I had verbally walked him out of the garden, I asked him what he had seen. He described in detail a rifle that his father had owned during World War I and had handed down to him. This one piece of information about the rifle opened up multiple opportunities to discuss his relationships with his two grown sons and the dilemma he currently faced about who should get this rifle. Over the next few months, he came to a decision to speak with his sons and ask them to share the rifle. Each agreed, possessing the rifle on alternating years.

Using the image of the rifle, this man became more aware of an issue that had been causing him much anxiety. He grew to enjoy the guided imagery sessions, and we continued to work together to build a trusting relationship. He even came to the painting classes I held and discovered that, although he had never painted before, he was able, as he called it, to "lose himself" or, as it is more commonly known in thematic arts programming, to be in "the flow."

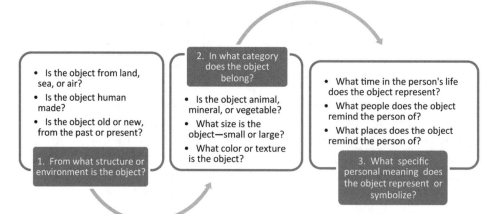

Figure 6.3.   Object relations theory can guide the use of conversation and themes in interactions during TTAP Method programming.

2. The semantic category to which the object belongs (animal, mineral, vegetable)

3. The specific personal meanings that the object represents (personal insight)

A person's ability to relate to an object from his or her life experience, to express its meaning(s) verbally or through such activities as sculpture (step 4), movement and dance (step 5), and drawing or painting (step 3), has positive effects on brain functioning and cognitive abilities (Brown, 1999). In step 1 (group conversation), the participants are engaged in a structured form of communication using an object or theme, which helps them to focus on the past, recall memories, and promote overall positive feelings of self-worth. In step 2 (music and meditation), participants, through guided imagery, can be taken to a safe, pleasant place in which to experience a notable object from their life experiences. Additionally, the structure of the TTAP Method can provide a focus over time that can ease the progression from a healthy, active state to a dependent state due to loss of memory, functional skills, and independence, all of which loom in the back of the mind of someone diagnosed with Alzheimer's.

THEME-CENTERED INTERACTION THEORY

Developed in the 1960s by German psychologist Ruth Cohn, *theme-centered interaction (TCI)* is a method and systematic model of working together and learning as a group (Hornecker, 2001). TCI focuses on the interrelationship between process, structure, and trust as mediating variables within the group learning experience. The interests of the individual participants, the group, and the theme (topic) must be in a dynamic balance (Figure 6.4). A group leader or moderator ensures that no one side dominates; rather, the individual-centered, group-centered, and theme-centered phases alternate. A theme is chosen in advance, relates to the experiences and interests of the participants, and is broad enough for the group to explore from the individual and group perspectives (Hornecker, 2001).

The TCI structure encompasses the following four components:

I (individual): The individual is motivated, shares interests, expands on personal histories, and experiences deeper levels of involvement with those in the group.

We (group): The group forms firm relationships in which trust and interpersonal bonds grow over time. The group dynamics foster learning through others and the "aha" concept of seeing something through another's point of view. Cooperation within the group is paramount for each participant to succeed, and thus cooperation is a natural structure for learning.

It (theme): The participants are much more apt to discuss subjects and themes in a group structure because of the non-threatening approach. No one person has control. Each is asked to participate in the discussion of what the topic or theme means personally and then to witness what it means to others in the group. This learning approach provides a richer dynamic because the content is viewed from a variety of individual perspectives.

Globe: The surrounding environment or context of the group experience, with its demands and constraints, is fundamental to the learning and development process of each participant. The globe is also represented by the group participants themselves (their experience, knowledge, strengths/weaknesses).

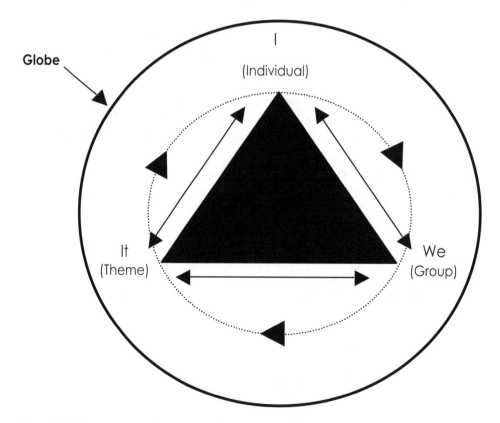

Figure 6.4. Theme-centered interaction structure and components.

Although Cohn's concepts were not developed for the Alzheimer's population, they fit well. Even someone with moderate Alzheimer's can start to feel more involved in the group as the others support and validate what he or she is sharing with the group. Discussions about values, insights, and life lessons are key factors in the process of personal development at any age, including for those with Alzheimer's. The TCI approach respects person-centered life experiences and the ability to evolve through the group process. This method is uniquely suited to integrate psychomotor and affective skills as part of the socialization process, which is currently lacking in many approaches to Alzheimer's care. '

Theme-Centered Interaction in the TTAP Method

The TTAP Method is based in part on the TCI approach; each session comprises a group, has a moderator or facilitator, and is developed around a theme. TCI as found in the TTAP Method integrates the individual into a group socialization setting in which the therapist guides participants in exploring a theme through creative arts activities. The therapist continually solicits input from the participants through conversation and art experiences. Each participant provides input from his or her personal life experiences, which the therapist incorporates into group programming. Each person has many opportunities for self-expression that the therapist can reinforce by giving repeated positive feedback. The entire group forms a close, trusting bond in the process.

As discussed in Chapter 2, the use of themes in creative arts programming has many benefits for the participants as well as for the therapist. Thinking in a thematic way allows the therapist to incorporate his or her own experiences into the programming while also sharing ideas from the group. The input of each person in the group is significant; the therapist encourages each participant to express individual thinking to promote interactions with others in the group and the sharing of self. An important goal for the therapist is to identify central themes that operate on different levels (individual, family, intergenerational, sociocultural) in order to develop effective therapeutic interactions, activities, and social events that will enhance social and personal connections for those with Alzheimer's (Papp & Imber-Black, 2004). Themes can also allow the group to discuss deeply personal topics that people with Alzheimer's are typically not asked about. Spiritual and end-of-life themes, for example, allow participants to give witness to how they are feeling. Successfully integrating themes of meaning and spirituality into end-of-life care can encourage dying people to find meaning and purpose in living, even up to the day of their passing. Themes may also reveal the needs of clients, including those with early-stage Alzheimer's, whose focus is on loss of memory, loss of self, and loss of life. Recognizing and understanding these needs can help the therapist choose responses that are appropriate and can serve therapeutic goals for the client at any stage of the disease process (Shapiro et al., 1999). (See Chapter 2 for a detailed discussion of the benefits of thematic programming.)

The structured thematic approach of the TTAP Method requires an active, participatory role by the therapist in leading group interactions around the chosen theme. In the TTAP Method, each step adds to defining who each participant is, each day of his or her life. A learning process is also continually stimulated in each step. In Step 1 (conversation), a theme allows people in the group to connect on a deep, meaningful level with others who are sharing their own experiences, particularly of loss of cognition, short-term memory, and so forth. In Step 2 (meditation or relaxation and guided imagery), the group is led down a path through a meditation, yet each individual will focus on, recall, and remember what he or she saw or experienced through the mind's eye. Sharing these memories has been shown to enhance verbalization, thus increasing participants' ability to be more aware of themselves and one another. With Step 3 (painting), Step 4 (sculpture), and Step 5 (movement and dance), individuals work autonomously and experience a self-respect for their work, their interpretations, and the social cohesiveness with the other group members that grows from the creative arts process (Levine Madori, 2007, 2009a,b,c). In Step 6 (poetry and storytelling), writing and the use of words in poems and stories enable participants to reflect deeply within and then be present for those in the group as each shares his or her writing, reinforcing interpersonal and intrapersonal experiences. In Step 7 (food programming) and Step 8 (theme event), participants show cultural respect and sensitivity while sharing their likes and dislikes, which enhances awareness of self and others. Food also establishes and reminds participants of rituals to be enjoyed and shared in a lively atmosphere, which encourages socialization. In Step 9 (phototherapy), the participants once again can learn about themselves and others in the safe context of the group. In taking pictures of each other, they feel a heightened sense of connectedness in responding to others and respecting the interpersonal relationships formed.

THEORY OF GEROTRANSCENDENCE

Developed in the 1990s by Swedish sociologist Lars Tornstam, gerotranscendence is defined as "the final stage in a possible natural progression toward maturation and wisdom" (Thornstam, 2005). According to the theory, a person experiences gerotranscendence later in life as a series of changes or developments that typically include a redefinition of the self and relationships to others. The characteristics of gerotranscendence include the following:

- A person becomes less self-absorbed and more selective in the choice of social and other activities.

- A person feels an increased affinity with past generations and a decreased interest in superfluous interactions.

- A person experiences a decreased interest in material things and a greater need for solitary meditation. Positive solitude becomes more important.

- There is also often a feeling of communion with the universe and a redefinition of time, space, life, and death (Tornstam, 2005).

This perspective goes directly against the prevailing belief that values and interests remain static as one ages and that aging means continuing to be the same person from middle age onward rather than achieving positive and meaningful self-actualization by retreating into one's own consciousness (Tornstam, 2005). Gerotranscendence is not a state of withdrawal or disengagement. Rather, Tornstam attributes the increased need for solitude as one ages, and for the company of only a few intimates, to continuing maturation. So an aging loved one is not necessarily self-isolating or deteriorating; he or she is continuing to self-evolve and mature, even later in life.

The theory of gerotranscendence is largely about the change and reconstruction of identity and personal frames of reference as a person ages. Through his research, Tornstam found that the phenomenon of gerotranscendence and the process of structured life review and reminiscence are intertwined. One must have structured opportunities to revisit the past with the wisdom one currently holds to engage in the critically important process of self-actualization. Life review and reminiscence can be used in ways other than that of stabilizing an already developed identity. Reminiscing with others and the ability to engage in structured life review provide the fundamental feedback from others that is needed to integrate past life experiences into who a person is at present (Tornstam, 1999).

How the TTAP Method Interprets the Theory of Gerotranscendence

The theory of gerotranscendence provides a framework by which older adults with dementia can be encouraged to actively engage in, disengage from, or reengage in social and other activities and relationships with others, as influenced by the events and experiences of their lives. Jung stated, "All true things must change and only that which changes remains true" (Jung, 1963). I believe this is the case even for individuals with Alzheimer's disease and other forms of dementias, who continue to change and evolve despite some degree of functional and cognitive deficits.

Consider how the TTAP Method interprets the four main principles of the theory of gerotranscendence:

1. *A person becomes less self-occupied and at the same time more selective in the choice of social and other activities.* In step 1 (group conversation), step 2 (music and meditation), and step 5 (movement and dance), the individual can choose to participate in activities that he or she finds engaging and enjoyable on a personal level. The sessions are not structured as typical activity conversation groups, in which, for example, discussion centers on a topic in the news. Rather, the TTAP Method is structured around whatever a person wants to share with the group participants, and the group actively values the personal nature of what is shared.

2. *A person feels an increased affinity with past generations and a decreased interest in superfluous social interaction.* In step 2 (music and meditation), step 6 (group writing experience), step 8 (theme event), and step 9 (phototherapy), the participant has the continual opportunity to revisit the past and the generations he or she has produced or descended from. The group writing experience, for example, encourages the individual to reflect on a theme in writing in the present time or in the past. A poem, short story, or letter-writing activity can be combined with phototherapy to share with loved ones. The themed event offers participants the opportunity to socialize in a structured event that continually draws from their past or present experiences and interests as well as strengths and abilities.

3. *A person might also experience a decreased interest in material things and a greater need for solitary meditation. Positive solitude becomes more important.* In step 2 (music and meditation), the individual is provided daily opportunities for structured relaxation and meditation. Participating in a meditation can promote feelings of union and comfort with the self on a level not previously attained for people with Alzheimer's. (For therapists unfamiliar with leading a meditation, one is included in Chapter 3 that can be used with people with Alzheimer's.)

4. *A person often feels communion with the universe and a redefinition of time, space, life, and death.* As discussed in Chapter 2, the TTAP Method promotes optimal experience, or being in the *flow*, which includes, among others, the following elements: a loss of time, deep concentration and focus, intense involvement, an intrinsically rewarding experience, and a transcendence of self. The ability of the TTAP Method to connect and engage the individual throughout the disease process enhances feelings of self-worth and self-respect as well as a sense of connection with not only the here and now, but also something greater, perhaps, with no boundaries between past, present, and future.

The TTAP Method encourages those with Alzheimer's to do the following:

- Engage socially, emotionally, and cognitively either within a group setting or one-on-one with the therapist

- Continue to explore the self and relationships with others in the care environment

- Apply those strengths and abilities that remain, thereby enhancing self-esteem, mood, memory, and use of language as well as affirming a sense of self that allows the individual to transcend the often self-perceived limitations of the disease.

THE LEVINE MADORI TAXONOMY: UNDERSTANDING THE PRINCIPLES AND PRACTICES OF THE TTAP METHOD

The previous sections outlined the various aging, developmental, and psychological theories that comprise the underpinnings of the TTAP Method. This section will further define the TTAP Method as a taxonomy, or classification, of learning and cognitive stimulation for people with Alzheimer's disease and other dementias.

In the United States during the late 1950s into the early 1970s, social psychologists attempted to dissect and classify the varied domains of human learning: *cognitive* (knowledge, development of intellectual skills); *affective* (feelings, values, appreciation, enthusiasms, motivations, attitudes); and *psychomotor* (physical movement, coordination, use of motor skills). The resulting efforts yielded a series of taxonomies in each area: Bloom's Taxonomy (1956) (cognitive domain), Krathwohl's Taxonomy (1964) (affective domain), and Harrow's Taxonomy (1972) (psychomotor domain). A *taxonomy* is a form of classification and is arranged hierarchically, proceeding from the simplest functions (recalling facts) to those that are more complex (evaluation) (Wilson, 2006).

The Levine Madori Taxonomy™ (2012) classifies the different ways that people with Alzheimer's and other dementias can learn and retain information through therapeutic art and recreation. It further identifies how cognitive functioning and ultimately quality and life, well-being, and self-esteem are enhanced for people with Alzheimer's through the TTAP Method by incorporating the concepts of the Continuum of Psychological Domains (physical, cognitive, social, emotional, spiritual), as well as the most common strengths and abilities an individual with Alzheimer's possesses throughout the disease process (CCDERS Approach™ [Chapter 2]).

Also included in the hierarchy of the Levine Madori Taxonomy are Bloom's six cognitive levels of complexity of thinking and learning (Chapter 5). In 2000, Anderson and Krathwohl condensed, expanded, and reinterpreted Bloom's Taxonomy. As shown in the comparison Figures 6.5 (A) and (B) of the original and revised versions, the six cognitive levels were changed from noun to verb form and their order was changed; the lowest level, *knowledge*, was renamed *remember*; *comprehension* was renamed *understanding*; and *synthesis* was moved to the highest level and changed to *create*. Anderson and Krathwohl defined the new categories of thinking and learning as follows (from lowest to highest level) (Anderson & Krathwohl, 2000):

Remember: Retrieving, recognizing, or recalling knowledge from memory to produce definitions, facts, or lists.

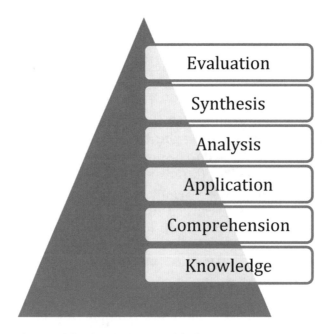

Figure 6.5 (A). Bloom's Taxonomy (1956).

Understand: Constructing meaning from different types of verbal, written, and graphic messages derived through interpreting, exemplifying, classifying, summarizing, inferring, comparing, or explaining.

Apply: Carrying out or using a procedure through execution or implementation. A person uses or applies learned material through models, presentations, interviews, or simulations.

Analyze: Breaking material or concepts into parts, determining how the parts relate or interrelate to one another or to an overall structure or purpose by differentiating, organizing, and attributing. A person analyzes material by creating charts, diagrams, or other graphic representations.

Evaluate: Making judgments based on criteria and standards by checking and critiquing. A person can use reports, recommendations, and so forth to demonstrate the process of evaluation.

Create: Putting elements together to form a coherent or functional whole; reorganizing elements into a new pattern or structure by generating, planning, or producing. Creating requires a person to put parts together in a new way or to synthesize parts into something new and different. This is the most difficult mental function in the revised Bloom's Taxonomy.

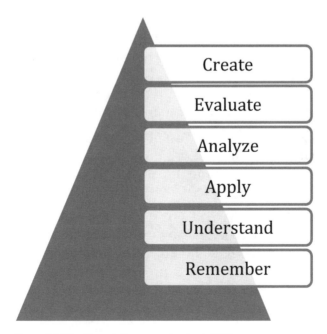

Figure 6.5 (B). Bloom's Taxonomy (revised, 2000).

Each level of Bloom's Taxonomy (2000) is represented in one or more of the steps of the TTAP Method, as follows:

Remembering in the TTAP Method: Participants recognize and recall relevant knowledge from their long-term memory, which is achieved through reminiscence around a chosen theme. The therapist uses graphic organization tools to focus the participants on the chosen theme and to assist them in remembering, including word lists, charts, graphs, and worksheets (group conversation [step 1]).

Understanding in the TTAP Method: For each of the steps, participants construct verbal, written, or graphical meaning by interpreting, classifying, summarizing, inferring, comparing, and explaining ideas and experiences based around a theme. With each step of the TTAP Method understanding is also derived by sharing with and bearing witness to others in the group.

Applying in the TTAP Method: Steps 3 through 11 of the TTAP Method are structured to assist the participants in carrying out or executing a procedure or process as part of a creative arts activity. Applying knowledge can be facilitated through role-playing (dance [step 5]), model-building (sculpture [step 4]), scrapbooking (drawing and painting [step 3]), collection and sharing of ideas (group conversation [step 1]), and so forth.

Analyzing in the TTAP Method: Participants break material into constituent parts, determining how they relate to one another and to the overall theme. This is done by organizing, differentiating, and attributing (group conversation [step 1]), as well as through feedback, assessment, and evaluation (step 12).

Evaluating in the TTAP Method: Participants form and express personal judgments and critiques at the end of each session of thematic programming through feedback, assessment, and evaluation (step 12).

Creating in the TTAP Method: For steps 3 through 11, participants piece materials together to form a coherent or functional whole or reorganize elements into a unique, personal pattern or structure. Each thematic programming session offers endless opportunities for participants to plan and create.

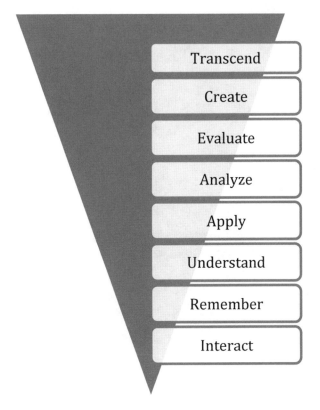

Figure 6.6. Levine Madori Taxonomy (2012), which includes Bloom's Taxonomy (2000).

The Levine Madori Taxonomy differs from Bloom's Taxonomy (2000) in the following ways in applying the TTAP Method to the Alzheimer's population (Figure 6.6):

- The inversion of the pyramid structure, representing the importance of actions or "doing," especially for those with Alzheimer's.

- The addition of *interact*, representing the significant and primary role the group interactions play in enhancing understanding, application, and creation.

- The addition of *transcendence* as the last (highest) layer in the pyramid structure, representing how empowered, self-confident, self-motivated, and emotionally fulfilled one can feel by engaging in the creative arts.

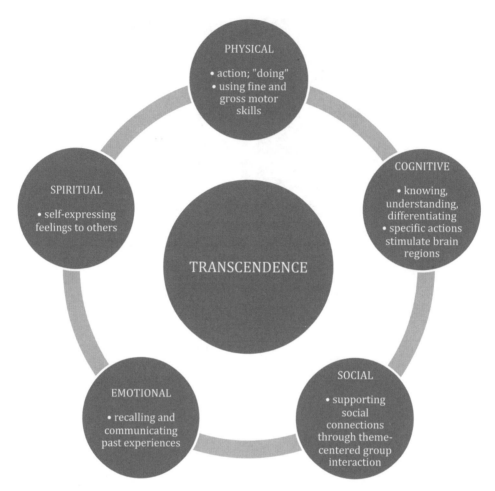

Figure 6.7. The Levine Madori Taxonomy incorporates the five psychological domains of self as well as a person's strengths and abilities, thereby empowering an individual to transcend the self-perceived limitations of dementia.

A dynamic thematic programming intervention that stimulates individuals diagnosed with Alzheimer's disease across the continuum of psychological domains opens up the possibility for personal growth, self-exploration, and emotional awareness through the group dynamic. This growth of moving forward, of going beyond what most people assume is possible for someone with dementia, is what I believe to be *transcendence* (Figure 6.7). Individuals with dementia living in long-term care, assisted living, and skilled nursing facilities are generally not expected to interact, recall, or give support to others. Use of the TTAP Method as a therapeutic intervention time and time again has proven through practice and research that, when given the opportunities to be engaged in thematic art and recreation activities, people with dementia can and do transcend what is expected of them as well as their own personal expectations.

CONCLUSION

As life expectancy is continually redefined and as the aging population grows larger, so too will new aging, developmental, and psychological perspectives emerge that must integrate the needs of older adults with Alzheimer's and other dementias. The role of the art and recreation therapist will become increasingly important in providing, through person-centered thematic programming, opportunities for this complicated process of integration to develop and unfold. Providing multiple opportunities to revisit the past, integrate the past with the present, and look into the future, the role of the creative arts and recreation therapist is central to the facilitation of psychological wellness and emotional fulfillment during the last stages of life for those with dementia. The TTAP Method creates an enriching environment for older adults with Alzheimer's and other dementias to enjoy this full expression of self and the many benefits that can result.

CHAPTER 7

Documentation and Replication of Research on the TTAP Method

This chapter looks at the available research on the effectiveness of the TTAP Method as an intervention for people with Alzheimer's disease and other dementias and discusses the need for more evidence-based methodologies that can generate reliable structure for and documentation of future research. The systematic nature of The TTAP Method® makes it highly replicable, which in turn makes it a valuable research tool for demonstrating the measurable benefits of using the creative arts and recreation therapy with this population. The TTAP Method provides new insight into what is happening during the arts and recreation therapy intervention by identifying which brain regions and functions are stimulated and which learning styles are used with each step in the TTAP Method. The documentation process that is part of the TTAP Method is valuable for several reasons. Not only does it demonstrate that creative arts programming directly improves a client's treatment outcome, but it can also be used to show monetary benefits to a care facility and increase opportunities for research. Using charts, graphs, and protocols, the therapist can provide structured documentation with respect to the scope, frequency, and duration of programming as well as to the person-centered nature of the intervention, thereby increasing the effectiveness of assessment and evaluation of treatment outcomes.

RESEARCH ON THE TTAP METHOD

To date, 11 studies (8 published) have assessed the effectiveness of the TTAP Method, and provide a structure and basis for the replication of research on the power of creative arts therapy in caring for people with Alzheimer's.

A study conducted in 2008 looked at 50 well-elderly individuals who regularly participated in activities at a community day center serving primarily a Spanish-speaking population. The participants were divided into two groups: a control group of 25 people who continued to participate in regular activities at the center and 25 people who participated in a 12-week, structured art therapy program based on the TTAP Method, with an hour-long art session each week. Study analysis showed positive and significant correlations to increased cognition and socialization in those who participated in the art therapy sessions compared with those who did not (Alders & Levine Madori, 2010).

The results of a second study that was conducted in 2008 and for which I was a principal investigator through the Cornell University Memory and Cognitive Screening Services were not statistically significant because of the small number of participants (eight). Of importance, however, were the written and videotaped personal evaluations and statements given by the participants every 3 weeks. The written questionnaires showed a marked correlation between perceived increase in cognition and attendance in the TTAP Method program. The participants also agreed to be interviewed by video camera after the tenth week, and all eight stated that they felt an increase in cognitive recall after participating in the programming.

For a study that was conducted in 2009 at Bergen Regional Medical Center in New Jersey, eight residents diagnosed with moderate to severe Alzheimer's and living in a secure dementia unit participated once a week in 2 hours of creative arts activities based on the TTAP Method for 8 successive weeks. The residents were asked to evaluate how they felt after each session. Results showed an increase in self-worth and self-esteem as well as a strong sense of having a voice because they had been asked to evaluate the programming. (See Appendix A for sample TTAP Method programming protocols.)

A 2010 study conducted at Northern Manor Geriatric Health Care Center in New York involved four residents who were diagnosed with Alzheimer's and living in a dementia care unit. The participants were asked questions to gauge their experiences of the art therapy sessions. The results indicated that they felt that the sessions were important and pleasurable and meaningfully added to their overall quality of life, even in the face of Alzheimer's (Levine Madori, et al., 2010). (The Northern Manor study is discussed further in this chapter under "Documenting Specific Treatment Outcomes from the TTAP Method.")

THE ROLE OF DOCUMENTATION IN CREATIVE ARTS THERAPIES

The Centers for Medicare and Medicaid Services provides coverage for health-related services to people age 65 or older and to people under the age of 65 with certain disabilities. Reimbursement for services is administered at the state level, with variations from state to state (Kane & Kane, 1981). Art and recreation therapy is included as a reimbursable service within the provisions for Partial Hospitalization for Geriatrics (American Art Therapy Association, 2007); however, states cover this service at different levels. The primary reason why art and recreation therapy are not universally covered by Medicare is because of the limited research and documentation within the fields as to their efficacy as care and treatment interventions (Eaton, Doherty, & Widrick, 2007). Increasing the type of standardized documentation, such as that offered through use of the TTAP Method, would contribute valuable data and efficacy measures that could lead to more funding opportunities to apply the method in caring for people with Alzheimer's and other forms of dementia, and could increase coverage of art and recreation therapy in general through Medicare.

DOCUMENTING SPECIFIC TREATMENT OUTCOMES FROM THE TTAP METHOD

Depending on the scope and goals of a research project, the impact of the TTAP Method can be measured in terms of cognitive performance, behavior changes, affect presentation, fall prevention, decreased agitation, engagement in programming, medication reduction, and language usage, among other treatment goals. Therapists can use the TTAP Method to facilitate specific therapeutic learning styles and treatment outcomes by establishing clear objectives that can be outlined and systematically evaluated as short- and long-term clinical goals. Furthermore, through such systematization, outcomes can be efficiently documented to foster collaboration between professionals from various specializations within the creative arts therapies (e.g., music, dance and movement, art, expressive arts, drama).

As the Alzheimer's population continues to grow and as state and federal governments are increasingly imposing stricter eligibility requirements for coverage, proper documentation is needed to assist in standardizing effective treatment and care interventions. Art and recreation therapists must have a hand in developing more reliable ways to assess, plan, implement, and evaluate the programming they provide on a daily basis. The sections that follow offer examples of specific treatment outcomes of the TTAP Method that can be measured.

Documentation of Session Attendance and Duration

Documentation of attendance for those diagnosed with Alzheimer's will enhance efficacy research studies and provide quality assurance that programming is being developed and implemented to best meet the needs of the participants (Figure 7.1) (Levine Madori et al., 2010).

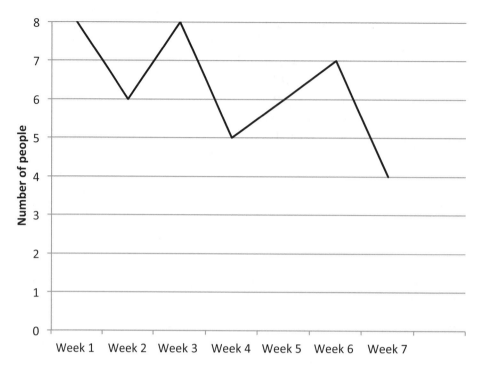

Figure 7.1. Attendance

Throughout the duration of a study the number of participants attending an art and recreation therapy session will vary. Within the TTAP Method structure, the therapist can easily document time, frequency, and duration for each participant.

Figure 7.1 shows the number of participants for each art therapy session for the Northern Manor study and the days for which attendance was lowest (i.e., first day of the month), which may allow for future programming planning. Moreover, attrition rates were analyzed to evaluate the quality of each session, the intrinsic motivation on the part of participants, and the appeal of the particular therapy provided.

Documentation of attendance is significant for several reasons. Current Medicare and Medicaid reimbursement policies require therapists to document attendance and time in programming to a greater degree than ever before in treating and caring for those with Alzheimer's. State and federal regulations (Medicare and Medicaid) require documentation in each resident's medical record of participation in specific activities and for what period of time. Charting patient or resident attendance can also be directly correlated to overall wellness and psychosocial well-being (Alders & Levine Madori, 2010; Levine Madori, 2009). Furthermore, previous guidelines for best practice have established that a therapeutic group should consist of no more than four participants per therapist (American Art Therapy Association, 2007). Therefore, charting the number of participants establishes programming quality for the population served. Finally, documentation contributes to a standardized approach to treatment using creative art and recreation therapies, thus systematically ensuring quality control.

Documentation of Person-Centered Care

Chapters 2 and 3 discuss the importance of engaging older adults with Alzheimer's and other forms of dementia in person-centered activities on a daily basis to stimulate the brain and thereby enhance cognition, verbal expression, and self-esteem. The first two steps of the TTAP Method (conversation [step 1] and music and meditation [step 2]) have been shown to immediately allow individuals with dementia to access and share significant memories from their past, which has a direct impact on their ability to socialize and form new relationships. For example, in the 2010 study conducted at Northern Manor Geriatric Center, participants were found to have naturally formed deep social relationships with those around them over the course of an 8-week program at the skilled nursing facility. This was due in part to the fact that TTAP Method sessions are unlike traditional activity programming in that the primary focus is the sharing and self-expression of long-term memories and life experiences (person-centered focus).

Other research studies in the United States as well as in Finland have shown that the TTAP Method provides many opportunities for enhanced verbal expression during creative arts therapy sessions, demonstrating that structured, formalized programming can be guided by the client as a form of person-centered care (Levine Madori, 2007; 2009a,b,c; Alders & Levine Madori, 2010). Qualitative data gathered from five Finnish studies reveal that researchers were consistently surprised by the depth of the verbal disclosures that occurred during the group sessions and the apparent risks that the participants took with one another (Hanski & Kahola, 2009; Ketola, 2010; Peltokangas & Rantala, 2009; Vanska, 2009). Participants even expressed genuine concern about whether sessions would continue, stating that they enjoyed the art and recreation activities. Treatment outcomes were shown to have improved based on the documentation of the range and intensity of emotional and verbal responses. Additional findings from five Finnish studies have shown that TTAP Method programming was significant in activating memories as well as stimulating mental personal images and positive conversations around the session theme. The sessions were also shown to have exercised remaining cognitive skills.

TTAP Method programming created enthusiasm among and creativity between residents, staff, and family members, thereby enhancing quality of life for the participants.

Documentation of Self-Perceived Quality of Life

Not until 2006 and then again in 2008 did researchers begin to ask residents what they needed and expected in therapeutic programming (Tabourne, Jung, & McClear, 2008; Woods et al., 2006). As part of the 2010 Northern Manor study of the efficacy of the TTAP Method, students from St. Thomas Aquinas College developed questions for session participants that were directed at measuring how the residents felt about the therapeutic programming. The questions focused on activity importance, personal perceived pleasure, level of interest in the activity, intensity of response, how personal the activity was to each resident, and how meaningful the session experience was.

At the end of each TTAP session the eight residents were asked to respond to the following questions using a scale from 0 to 5 (0 being the lowest and 5 the highest):

1. Did this activity make you feel bored at any time?

2. Are you looking forward to next week's session?

3. Does the meditation quiet your mind?

4. Are you in good spirits during this session?

5. Does this session take your mind off the future?

6. Did you feel restless or fidgety during this session?

7. Did this session help your memory?

8. Did this session add excitement to your life?

9. On a scale of 1 to 5, did this session increase your energy or make you more aware?

The students then categorized and developed a subset using these questions for the following variables:

Quality of life (1, 5, 8)

Mood (2, 4, 5, 6)

Relaxation (3)

Anxiety (6)

Memory and cognition (7)

Physical stamina (6, 9)

In reviewing the results of the study, it is important to identify its weaknesses and strengths. Note that documented responses were collected only through week 7 because a formal session was not held on the last day for week 8. The weaknesses of the study include the lack of a control group or experimental group to measure and compare the same variables against the traditional therapeutic setting. Additionally, the sessions were conducted over a short period of 8 weeks rather than for 6 months or longer. The primary goal, however, was simply to give the residents a voice to express how they felt about participating in the activities and how the group sessions were affecting their day. The ability to give people diagnosed with Alzheimer's opportunities to engage in social groups that encourage and support communication, sharing, and intrinsic motivation is paramount to changing the culture of care in the United States.

It is significant to note that many of the residents in this study verbalized disappointment when they were told at week 5 that the sessions were going to end in 3 weeks. They were very upset that the special sessions would soon come to an end. They said that this type of programming should be done regularly. The meditations, in particular, were something new to them. This activity gave them the chance to relax and clear their minds, made them feel better, and provided them with the time and opportunity to recall and share memories they had not thought about in years.

Figures 7.2–7.7 show the study results for quality of life, mood, meditation and relaxation, anxiety, memory and cognition, and physical stamina.

Quality of Life. For question 1 (Did this activity make you feel bored at any time?), the boredom level was at its highest in the first week for the first session because the activities were new to the residents. As the sessions continued over the 7 weeks, residents expressed feeling less bored. Resident responses to question 5 (Does this session take your mind off the future?) averaged a score of 3.7 for the first session, a healthy number considering how new the activities were to them. As the weeks progressed, residents averaged a 4.8 for their responses to question 5, a clear indication that the activities helped take their minds off of the future by focusing their attention on the tasks at hand. For question 8 (Did this session add excitement to your life?), residents had a very high average of nearly 4 through session 4, and it reached a high of 5 by session 5. The steady drop in the responses to this question for the last three sessions reflects the fact that, as mentioned earlier, residents were feeling disappointment at learning in week 5 that the sessions would be ending in 3 more weeks.

Question 1: Did this activity make you feel bored at any time?
Question 5: Does this session take your mind off the future?
Question 8: Did this session add excitement to your life?

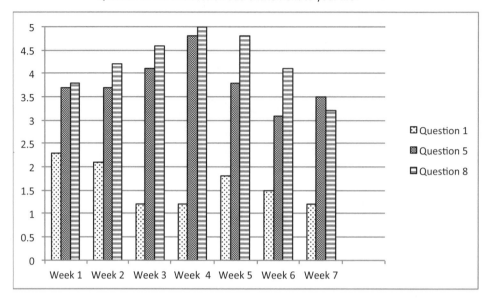

Figure 7.2. Quality of llife

Question 2: Are you looking forward to next week's session? *Question 4:* Are you in good spirits during this session?
Question 5: Does this session take your mind off the future? *Question 6:* Did you feel restless or fidgety during this session?

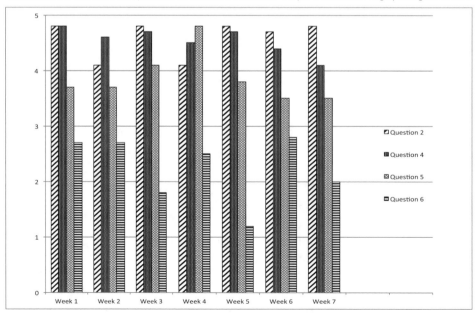

Figure 7.3. Mood

Question 3: Does the meditation quiet your mind?

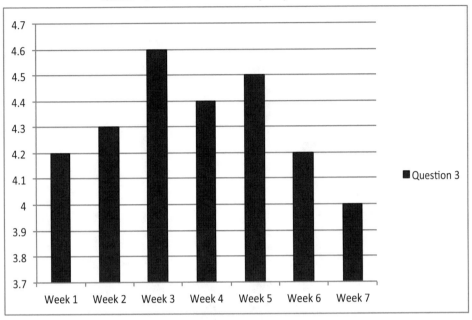

Figure 7.4. Meditation and relaxation

Mood. For questions 2 and 4 (Are you looking forward to next week's session? Are you in a good spirits during this session?), resident responses averaged high, between 4 and 5. Responses to question 5 initially averaged 3.7, as noted above, and rose to 4.8 as the weeks progressed. Clearly the activities helped take residents' minds off of negativity and let them focus and engage their attention on the positive aspects of their day. For question 6 (Did you feel restless or fidgety during this session?), residents averaged a low rate of feeling fidgety or restless during the 7 weeks, an indication that in general they felt comfortable participating in the activities. Their minds were also less likely to wander if they were focused on an activity.

Meditation and Relaxation. Each week a different student led the meditation to begin the session. In the first 2 weeks, the meditation was in a room where the residents were easily distracted. In the third week, the participants were moved to a different room with fewer distractions. Their responses to question 3 (Does the meditation quiet your mind?) were on average higher following the room change. This highlights the key role the environment plays in providing programming that is uninterrupted and without distractions. In week 6, the

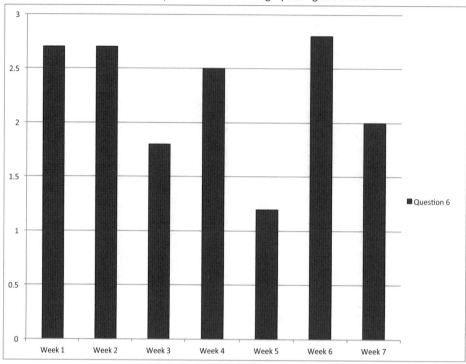

Figure 7.5. Anxiety

residents were aware that the sessions would be ending, and a reduction in relaxation can be seen, which can be attributed in part to the stress of knowing that the sessions would not continue much longer.

Anxiety.   As has already been mentioned with respect to meditation and relaxation, residents reported a low rate of feeling fidgety or restless during the 7 weeks in response to question 6 (Did you feel restless or fidgety during this session?), which indicates a lack of anxiety and stress in participating in the activities. A score of 2.5 was the highest seen during the 8 weeks. Participants may have felt less fidgety during particular activities.

Memory and Cognition.   For question 7 (Did this session help your memory?), the scores ranged from 3.7 to 4.3, confirming that the residents were able to judge for themselves the activities' effects on their cognitive abilities. The lowest score was after session 4, which involved

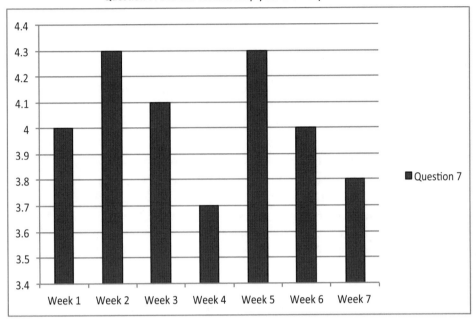

Question 7: Did this session help your memory?

Figure 7.6. Memory and cognition

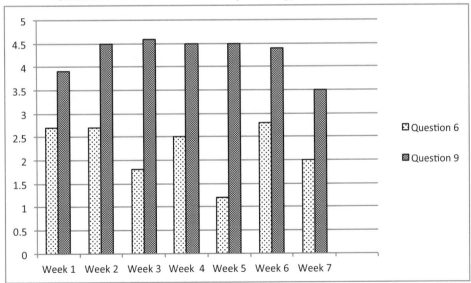

Question 6: Did you feel restless or fidgety during this session?
Question 9: Did this session increase your energy or make you more aware?

Figure 7.7. Physical stamina

decorating a mirror. The lower score, however, may have been in response to the actual activity. The residents actively engaged in looking at their reflections, and during the session the students documented negative comments from residents who saw themselves as old. This particular skilled nursing facility has few mirrors because residents with memory loss can become confused by seeing their reflection. This activity revealed another reason for minimizing the use of mirrors, in that the residents did not appear to enjoy the use of reflections.

Physical stamina.   For question 9 (Did this session increase your energy or make you more aware?), the residents' energy levels were high during each of the seven sessions. Interesting to note is that restlessness (question 6) was at its documented highest score during session 6. It was during this session that residents started verbalizing their feelings about having this program end; signs of restlessness were evident in their responses.

Documentation of Brain Regions Stimulated

In documenting their results, the students conducting the Northern Manor study also identified for each session which brain regions were stimulated. Brain illustrations were commissioned with the targeted stimulated areas highlighted (Figures 7.8, 7.9). A table can also be created to document which brain regions were stimulated for each programming directive, as well as any positive participant commentary associated with each step of the TTAP Method (Table 7.1). (See

Table 7.1. Sample documentation of brain regions stimulated during TTAP Method programming.

Programming	TTAP Method steps	Positive participant commentary	Brain region(s) stimulated
Music and meditation	1,2	I felt free during this group.	Broca's area, Temporal lobe
Oil pastel drawing	1,2,3	I feel very happy.	Broca's area, Parietal lobe, Temporal lobe
Wreath sculpture	1,2,4	I was able to really create something.	Broca's area, Cerebellum, Motor cortex, Temporal lobe
Mask-making	1,2,4	I was able to do what I wanted.	Broca's area, Cerebellum, Motor cortex, Temporal lobe
Memory box	1,2,4	Someone saved me a lot of trouble.	Broca's area, Cerebellum, Motor cortex, Temporal lobe
Painting	1,2,3	I am more active in this program.	Broca's area, Parietal lobe, Temporal lobe
Food event	1,2,7	I am always active.	Broca's area, Sensory cortex, Reticular formation, Temporal lobe

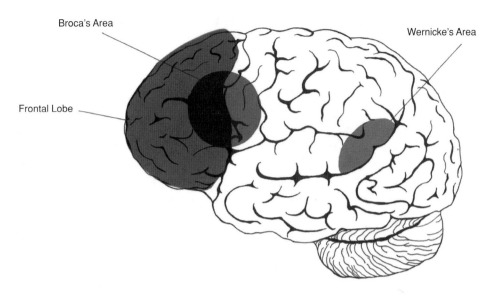

Figure 7.8.   Illustration of brain regions stimulated as part of a sculpture program (step 4). (Illustration by Lea Madori.)

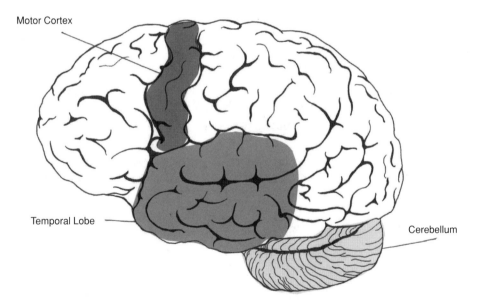

Figure 7.9.   Illustration of brain regions stimulated as part of a group writing experience program (step 6). (Illustration by Lea Madori.)

also Table 5.3 in Chapter 5, which lists the learning styles incorporated into each programming session of the Bergen Regional Medical Center study of the TTAP Method.)

Documentation of Monetary Impact on Facility

In 2009, I conducted a TTAP Method Certification Training Course at Linden Oaks of Edward Hospital in Chicago for all staff on the Gero-Psychiatric Unit working with patients diagnosed with moderate to severe Alzheimer's. Staff were trained and certified in the concepts of the TTAP Method as a way to structure programming for and interaction with patients. Several significant findings emerged when the outcomes of implementing the themed programming model were measured. Disruptive, aggressive, and emotional behaviors as well as the rate of falls decreased so much that the hospital projected it had saved more than $160,000 in nursing supervision in a 12-month period. Second, interactions among staff members and staff morale improved significantly, which led directly to the creation of more interdisciplinary programs for the patients. One of the continual struggles in moving from a medical model to a social model of care is the need for practitioners from different disciplines (nursing, certified nursing assistants, social workers) to work together to provide art and recreation activities. The TTAP Method provides different disciplines the tools they need to offer programming that is more intimate, emotional, and gratifying for clients and staff alike. Other similar research on the use of the TTAP Method in the United States and Finland supports an important outcome: Staff members feel more satisfied with their interactions with residents during the activities, which directly motivated them to develop more interactions and furthered an increase in the number of programs that the staff designed and led.

In the Linden Oaks study, nursing staff and certified nursing assistants were documented to have held more group creative arts activities than ever before in the Gero-Psychiatric Unit. Formal feedback gathered by hospital staff from patients showed positive responses to the programming, with one key response often noted: "Patient states that he or she feels ownership in the process of developing a themed activity."

CONCLUSION

In addition to providing therapists with the tools to plan and replicate interventions for future clients, the documentation aspects of the TTAP Method establish a structure and basis for the replication of research on the effectiveness of creative arts therapy in caring for people with Alzheimer's. Studies on the use of the TTAP Method have shown improved cognition, increased participation and time spent in programming, enhanced feelings of well-being, decreased isolation (increased social interactions), and so forth in people with dementia who are receiving care in adult day centers, assisted living communities, and skilled nursing facilities. Much more research is needed to foster national and international support for the necessity of creative arts programming as a method of improving quality of life and making the most of the remaining strengths and abilities of people with Alzheimer's and other forms of dementia. Through a structured documentation approach and more efficacy research, including interdisciplinary research, creative arts and recreation therapies can rise to the forefront of public awareness as effective interventions in caring for and interacting with people with dementia. Such awareness can lead to positive changes in the culture of care for those with mild, moderate, and advanced stages of Alzheimer's.

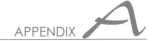
Program Protocols for the TTAP Method

Tapping into Creativity

PROGRAM PROTOCOL 1: WEEK/SESSION 1

TTAP Method Steps

Group conversation (step 1)
Music and meditation (step 2)

Treatment Protocol

Using music as part of group conversation and meditation/guided imagery

Materials

Two or three pieces of thematic music
CD player, tape player, or digital media player

Rationale

Guided imagery is a way in which to calm the mind and allow thoughts, both past and present, to surface. Using music, the therapist (group leader) speaks slowly to the residents, first relaxing the body and then the mind, while they are contemplating the sounds of the music. This exercise allows residents to freely access their long-term memory; listening to the music evokes mental images based around the chosen theme (summer). Once the participants have completed the guided imagery, the therapist leads a group discussion of what images were brought to mind for each person. Residents freely share in detailed language past experiences of summer. Reminiscing helps the individuals review positive and significant experiences they have had over the course of a lifetime. This group experience instills a sense of overall positive well-being and stimulates social and verbal interactions.

Referrals

This program is designed specifically for individuals diagnosed with mild Alzheimer's disease. Referrals to this program can be made through staff, social workers, and family members.

Risk Management

This program does not present any organizational risk. When reviewing memories, however, there is the concern that a participant may relive a negative or bad experience. Additionally, there might be memories that are too personal to share with the entire group. The recreation therapist must be aware of each participant's responses and be ready to support, comfort, or control any sad or uncomfortable memories that might arise.

Structure of Session

The music and meditation (guided imagery) should be no longer than 10 minutes. This will allow residents to become familiar with listening to music and allowing images to come into the "mind's eye" (e.g., sounds of the surf, summer theme; sounds of a tropical forest, animal theme; sound of wind, autumn theme). The process of becoming familiar with guided imagery is very common and usually takes one or two sessions for the participants to get used to. After the residents have listened to the music, start a conversation with open-ended questions. The length of the group conversation can range from 25 minutes to a full hour, including listening to the music.

Time Duration: 5 minutes

Introductions of group participants and group leader

Time Duration: 5 minutes

The therapist presents the goals of the session to the participants as follows:

- The therapist explains the importance of mental stimulation through music and meditation/guided imagery (body relaxation).

- The group will listen to music that will bring mental images to mind.

- The group will be encouraged to reminisce about past, present, and future experiences recalled through the guided imagery.

- The experiences/memories brought to mind through the guided imagery will be used to create art.

Time Duration: 10 minutes

Participants are invited to sit and listen to music with a summer theme.

Time Duration: 15–30 minutes

The therapist leads the participants in conversation about what experiences/memories the music brought to mind, using a whiteboard, large poster board, or other graphic organizing tool to list the ideas and words based on the theme of summer.

The therapist asks the participants questions, such as the following:

When you were listening to the music, what were you thinking about?

Did you see a summer scene?

Were you concentrating on the sounds?

What sounds could be heard?

What did those sounds remind you of?

Did any memories come to you while you were listening to the music?

Process Criteria

The group leader will never leave residents unattended. If any one of the group members becomes agitated or upset, another staff member should immediately take the person out of the group. The leader will continually encourage quiet listening during the music and conversation after the music is heard.

The *Therapist* will

Set up the CD player, tape player, or digital media player

Instruct residents on how to "listen" to music, with or without eyes closed

Comfort residents who might be in need

Encourage discussion of the music theme

Outcome Criteria

Residents will readily access memories of past experiences. The increased socialization throughout the group should be noticeable. This experience allows individuals who normally would not share in conversation to do so through reminiscence and positive sharing experiences within a group.

The *Resident* will be able to

Express ideas or thoughts about the music (although he or she may need some encouragement from the therapist)

Socialize within the group around the chosen theme

Contribute to what is recorded by the group leader

Have multiple opportunities to reflect on the past and share feelings, accomplishments, and interests with the group

Credentialing

This program should be supervised by Certified Therapeutic Recreation Specialists (CTRS) and conducted by group leaders who have been trained.

Bibliography

BrainSkills. Vered, M. (November, 2010). Meditation. http://www.brainskills.co.uk/Meditation.html

St. Louis Public Library staff. (2010). Meditation for stress relief. http://www.slpl.org/slpl/interests/article240081100.asp

Yahoo Music. (December, 2005). Why music stimulates the human brain: The many faces of music. http://www.associatedcontent.com/article/17049/why_music_stimulates_the_human_brain.html

CNN.com. (December, 2000). Mind over matter: Meditation helps ease pain for some patients. http://archives.cnn.com/2000/HEALTH/alternative/09/04/meditation.pain.wmd/index.html

PROGRAM PROTOCOL 2: WEEK/SESSION 2

TTAP Method Steps

Group conversation (step 1)
Music and meditation (step 2)
Drawing and painting (step 3)

Treatment Protocol

Using memories from group conversation and meditation/guided imagery to create a thematic painting

Materials

Two or three pieces of thematic music
CD player, tape player, or digital media player
Large painting paper (18 × 24 inch)
Tempera paints, nontoxic (no more than six colors)
Cups for paints and water
Brushes

Rationale

Working from the ideas that were shared in the first session (based on the theme of summer), the therapist will lead the group in a thematic painting activity. Art helps residents to express their emotions and show creativity. The themes evoked through music encourage relaxation and enhance the residents' ability to recall long-term memories that are still very accessible in the initial stages of Alzheimer's. Researchers have found that art is a way to restore and even add to one's self-identity as well as to help individuals interpret images for problem solving, conflict, and resolution in the last stages of life.

Referrals

This program is designed specifically for individuals with mild Alzheimer's disease. Referrals to this program can be made through staff, social workers, and family members.

Risk Management

This program does not present any organizational risk. When reviewing memories, however, there is the concern that a participant may relive a negative or bad experience. Additionally, there might be memories that are too personal to share with the entire group. The recreation therapist must be aware of each participant's responses and be ready to support, comfort, or control any sad or uncomfortable memories that might arise.

Structure of Session

The therapist will lead the participants through the guided imagery used in the first session to refocus them on the chosen theme (summer). This second session will revisit the themes that emerged during the first session by looking at the white board or poster board that the therapist used to collect ideas and words from the participants. Residents will be given painting paper and asked to paint images or scenes that came to mind and were shared during the first session. Selection of nontoxic, water-soluble colored paints should be limited to no more than six colors to avoid frustration with choice.

Time Duration: 5 minutes

Introductions of group participants and group leader

Time Duration: 5 minutes

The therapist presents the goals of the session to the participants as follows:

- The therapist explains the importance of mental stimulation through music and meditation/guided imagery (body relaxation).
- The group will listen to music that will bring mental images to mind.
- The group will be encouraged to reminisce about past, present, and future experiences recalled through the guided imagery.
- The experiences/memories brought to mind through the guided imagery will be used to paint a scene or image.

Time Duration: 10 minutes

Participants are invited to sit and listen to music with a summer theme.

Time Duration: 5–10 minutes (or until the conversation subsides)

The therapist asks the participants questions, such as the following:

When you were listening to the music, what summer memory were you thinking about?

What did you remember?

Where were you?

Who was with you, if anyone?

What did the sounds of the music remind you of?

How does it make you feel thinking and reminiscing about this special memory, while listening to the music?

Time Duration: 20–30 minutes

Participants each get a piece of painting paper and will have the option of choosing which colors to use to create their thematic painting.

Process Criteria

The group leader will never leave residents unattended. If any one of the group members becomes agitated or upset, the person should be immediately taken out of the group by another staff member. The group leader will continually encourage the residents to paint while listening to quiet music in the background.

The *Therapist* will

Set up the CD player, tape player, or digital media player

Instruct residents on how to use the paints (demonstration)

Encourage discussion of the final project

Clean up and organize all supplies

Outcome Criteria

Residents will be reminded of the first session, accessing once again the memories of past experiences. Residents will create a painting to their satisfaction.

The *Resident* will

Be encouraged to remember thoughts and ideas shared during the first session

Have multiple opportunities to use fine motor coordination

Demonstrate or express feelings of accomplishment

Share thoughts, feelings, and his or her project with others

Reflect on the past

Reflect on positive memories through the art process

Credentialing

This program should be supervised by Certified Therapeutic Recreation Specialists (CTRS) and conducted by group leaders who have been trained.

Bibliography

BrainSkills. Vered, M. (November, 2010). Meditation. http://www.brainskills.co. uk/Meditation.html

St. Louis Public Library staff. (2010). Meditation for stress relief. http://www.slpl. org/slpl/interests/article240081100.asp

Yahoo Music. (December, 2005). Why music stimulates the human brain: The many faces of music. http://www.associatedcontent.com/article/17049/why_music_stimulates_the_human_brain.html

Karolinska Institutet. (February, 2009). Cognitive training can alter biochemistry of the brain. http://www.sciencedaily.com/releases/2009/02/090206081507.htm

PROGRAM PROTOCOL 3: WEEK/SESSION 3

TTAP Method Steps

Group conversation (step 1)
Music and meditation (step 2)
Sculpture (step 4)

Treatment Protocol

Using memories from group conversation and meditation/guided imagery to create a thematic floral centerpiece.

MATERIALS

Two or three pieces of thematic music
CD player, tape player, or digital media player
Colored tissue paper, nontoxic (no more than six colors)
Ready-made tissue flowers
Leaves
Glue

Rationale

This program uses a peer setting to enhance socialization, reinforce a previous thematic art experience, and stimulate cognitive abilities. Additionally, the participants will explore and use objects and materials that, through a thematic approach, encourage self-expression in a nonthreatening, shared group experience. The very act of tapping into one's inner resources empowers each resident while promoting feelings of mastery and increased self-esteem. The ability to make something out of raw materials is an enjoyable act at any age. This group experience enhances memory, orientation, and communication on many levels. The group leader stimulates orientation by continually linking activities. Stimulation of memories is continual as the group leader uses open-ended questions while residents are involved in the sculpture activity. Each resident will create a beautiful summer floral centerpiece to display in his or her room or to use as part of a future theme event (step 8) or drama or theater experience (step 11).

Referrals

This program is designed specifically for individuals with mild Alzheimer's disease. Referrals to this program can be made through staff, social workers, and family members.

Risk Management

This program does not present any organizational risk. When reviewing memories, however, there is the concern that a participant may relive a negative or bad experience. Additionally, there might be memories that are too personal to share with the entire group. The recreation therapist must be aware of each participant's responses and be ready to support, comfort, or control any sad or uncomfortable memories that might arise. All art materials are nontoxic and safe.

Structure of Session

The therapist will lead the participants through the guided imagery used in the first session to refocus them on the chosen theme (summer). This third session will revisit the themes that emerged during the first session by looking at the white board or poster board that the therapist used to collect ideas and words from the participants. Participants will be shown a finished floral centerpiece, which they each will then create. Each resident will be given a ready-made tissue flower and a selection of leaves and colored tissue paper (which will be limited to six colors to avoid frustration with choice).

Time Duration: 5 minutes

Introductions of group participants and group leader

Time Duration: 5 minutes

The therapist presents the goals of the session to the participants as follows:

- The therapist explains the importance of mental stimulation through music and meditation/guided imagery (body relaxation).

- The group will listen to music that will bring mental images to mind.

- The group will be encouraged to reminisce about past, present, and future experiences recalled through the guided imagery.

- Reflecting on what was seen during the guided imagery, each resident will create a summer floral centerpiece.

Time Duration: 10 minutes

Participants are invited to sit and listen to music with a summer theme.

Time Duration: 5–10 minutes (or until the conversation subsides)

The therapist asks the participants questions, such as the following:

When you were listening to the music, what summer images or scenes came to mind and what were you thinking about?

What did you remember?

What colors came to mind?

Who was with you, if anyone?

What did the sounds of the music remind you of?

How does it make you feel thinking and reminiscing about this special memory, while listening to the music?

Time Duration: 20–30 minutes

Participants will receive a ready-made tissue flower and will have the option of choosing from leaves and colored tissue paper to attach to its stem using glue.

Process Criteria

The group leader will never leave residents unattended. If any one of the group members becomes agitated or upset, the person should be immediately taken out of the group by another staff member. The group leader will continually encourage stimulating conversation during the activity and the use of fine motor coordination.

The *Therapist* will

Set up the CD player, tape player, or digital media player

Revisit and reflect on the first session

Hand out materials to each resident

Demonstrate how to make a flower using the colored tissue paper and glue

Demonstrate how to decorate the ready-made tissue flower

Encourage discussion of the final project

Clean up and organize all supplies

Outcome Criteria

Residents will be encouraged to recall what happened in the first session, reflect again on past experiences, and socialize with others in the group. Residents will be encouraged to create, with assistance, a floral centerpiece to be used in a future session.

The *Resident* will

Be encouraged to recall thoughts and ideas shared during the first session

Socialize with others about the self or the project

Have multiple opportunities to use fine motor coordination

Demonstrate or express feelings of accomplishment

Share thoughts, feelings, and his or her project with others

Reflect on positive memories through the art process

Credentialing

This program should be supervised by Certified Therapeutic Recreation Specialists (CTRS) and conducted by group leaders who have been trained.

Bibliography

BrainSkills. Vered, M. (November, 2010). Meditation. http://www.brainskills.co.uk/Meditation.html

St. Louis Public Library staff. (2010). Meditation for stress relief. http://www.slpl.org/slpl/interests/article240081100.asp

Yahoo Music. (December, 2005). Why music stimulates the human brain: The many faces of music. http://www.associatedcontent.com/article/17049/why_music_stimulates_the_human_brain.html

PROGRAM PROTOCOL 4: WEEK/SESSION 4

TTAP Method Steps

Group conversation (step 1)
Music and meditation (step 2)
Sculpture (step 4)

Treatment Protocol

Using memories from group conversation and meditation/guided imagery to create a thematic floral wreath.

Materials

Two or three pieces of thematic music
CD player, tape player, or digital media player
Artificial (nontoxic) or real flowers
Floral arrangements
Wreaths

Rationale

At the end of the floral centerpiece session, the participants asked to have another session using flowers. This is an example of how the TTAP Method promotes personal choice and the intrinsic motivation to participate in a group activity. As with each session, music is incorporated to stimulate thoughts and feelings long forgotten. Knowledge of music and its positive effects on people with Alzheimer's disease is continually growing. Clinical studies document the fact that individuals who can no longer recognize loved ones can still recall music of their generation (Cash, 2006). A study in Barcelona, Spain, found that 14 residents with mild Alzheimer's disease improved in social and emotional areas after receiving music therapy (Brotons & Marti, 2003). This program uses a peer setting to enhance socialization, reinforce a previous thematic art experience, and stimulate cognitive abilities. Additionally, the participants will explore and use objects and materials that, through a thematic approach, encourage self-expression in a nonthreatening, shared group experience. The residents will create a beautiful floral door wreath to hang from the front door of their room.

Referrals

This program is designed specifically for individuals with mild Alzheimer's disease. Referrals to this program can be made through staff, social workers, and family members.

Risk Management

This program does not present any organizational risk. When reviewing memories, however, there is the concern that a participant may relive a negative or bad experience. Additionally, there might be memories that are too personal to share with the entire group. The recreation therapist must be aware of each participant's responses and be ready to support, comfort, or control any sad or uncomfortable memories that might arise. All art materials are nontoxic and safe.

Structure of Session

The therapist will lead the participants through the guided imagery used in the first session to refocus them on the chosen theme (summer). This fourth session will revisit the themes that emerged during the first session by looking at the white board or poster board that the therapist used to collect ideas and words from the participants. The residents will be encouraged to share their experiences, thoughts, or concerns related to the previous week's session. They will be asked about how they are feeling about the sessions thus far (the activities and the outcomes). The participants will be shown a finished floral wreath. Each resident will then be given a wreath to decorate. Participants will choose from a selection of artificial or real flowers and ready-made floral arrangements to decorate their own wreath.

Time Duration: 5 minutes
Introductions of group participants and group leader

Time Duration: 5 minutes
The therapist discusses the goals of the session to the participants as follows:

- The therapist explains the importance of mental stimulation through music and meditation/guided imagery (body relaxation).

- The group will listen to music that will bring mental images to mind.

- The group will be encouraged to reminisce about past, present, and future experiences recalled through the guided imagery.

- Reflecting on what was seen during the guided imagery, each resident will create a floral wreath.

Time Duration: 10 minutes

Participants are invited to sit and listen to music with a summer theme.

Time Duration: 5–10 minutes (or until the conversation subsides)

The therapist asks the participants questions, such as the following:

When you were listening to the music, what summer images or scenes came to mind and what were you thinking about?

What did you remember?

What colors came to mind?

Who was with you, if anyone?

What did the sounds of the music remind you of?

How does it make you feel thinking and reminiscing about this special memory, while listening to the music?

Time Duration: 20–30 minutes

Participants will receive a wreath and will have the option of choosing from artificial or real flowers to decorate it with.

Process Criteria

The group leader will never leave residents unattended. If any one of the group members is getting agitated or upset, he or she should be immediately taken out of the group by another staff member. The group leader will continually encourage stimulating conversation during the activity and the use of fine motor coordination.

The *Therapist* will

Set up the CD player, tape player, or digital media player

Revisit and reflect on the first session

Hand out a wreath to each resident

Demonstrate how to decorate the wreath using artificial or real flowers

Encourage discussion of the final project

Clean up and organize all supplies

Outcome Criteria

Residents will be encouraged to recall what happened in the first session, reflect again on past experiences, and socialize with others in the group. Residents will be encouraged to create, with assistance, a floral wreath to be used in a future session.

The *Resident* will

Be encouraged to recall thoughts and ideas shared during the first session

Socialize with others about the self or the project

Have multiple opportunities to use fine motor coordination

Demonstrate or express feelings of accomplishment

Share thoughts, feelings, and his or her project with others

Reflect on positive memories through the art process

Credentialing

This program should be supervised by Certified Therapeutic Recreation Specialists (CTRS) and conducted by group leaders who have been trained.

Bibliography

BrainSkills. Vered, M. (November, 2010). Meditation. http://www.brainskills.co.uk/Meditation.html

St. Louis Public Library staff. (2010). Meditation for stress relief. http://www.slpl.org/slpl/interests/article240081100.asp

Yahoo Music. (December, 2005). Why music stimulates the human brain: The many faces of music. http://www.associatedcontent.com/article/17049/why_music_stimulates_the_human_brain.html

TTAP Method Activity Assessment Form

Name of program _____

Give a brief description of activity, including any adaptive needs:

_____

_____

_____

_____

_____

_____

_____

_____

_____

_____

_____

_____

_____

_____

_____

_____

Population served _____

Ideal number of participants in group _____

BRAIN ASPECTS

Brain regions stimulated in this therapeutic activity:

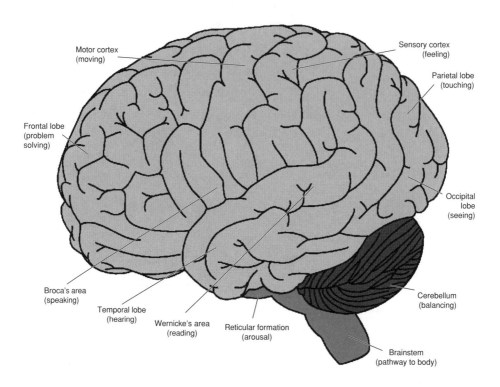

Which brain regions are stimulated during this program?

_____ Frontal lobe	_____ Wernicke's area
_____ Parietal lobe	_____ Broca's area
_____ Occipital lobe	_____ Cerebellum
_____ Temporal lobe	_____ Reticular formation
_____ Motor cortex	_____ Hippocampus
_____ Sensory cortex	_____ Entorhinal cortex

LEARNING ASPECTS

Check which learning style this activity encompasses (activity can encompass more than one learning style):

_____ Linguistic learner (the word player)

_____ Logical learner (the questioner)

_____ Spatial learner (the visualizer)

_____ Musical learner (the music lover)

_____ Kinesthetic learner (the mover)

_____ Interpersonal learner (the socializer)

_____ Intrapersonal learner (the individual)

PHYSICAL ASPECTS

1. What is the primary body position required?

    _____ prone   _____ kneeling

    _____ sitting   _____ standing

    other:_____

2. Which parts of the body are required?

    _____ arms   _____ legs

    _____ hands   _____ feet

    _____ head   _____ upper torso

    _____ neck   _____ lower torso

3. Which types of movement does this activity require?

    _____ bending   _____ skipping

    _____ catching   _____ reaching

    _____ stretching   _____ hopping

    _____ throwing   _____ grasping

    _____ standing   _____ running

    _____ hitting   _____ punching

    _____ walking

Coordination between parts and movement:

1   2   3   4   5

Low   High

Eye–hand coordination:

1   2   3   4   5

Low   High

Strength:

1   2   3   4   5

Low   High

Speed:

1   2   3   4   5

Low   High

Endurance:

1   2   3   4   5

Low   High

Energy:

1   2   3   4   5

Low   High

Flexibility:

1   2   3   4   5

Little   Much

Degree of cardiovascular activity involved:

1   2   3   4   5

Little   Much

SOCIAL ASPECTS

Interaction pattern regarding person and object (check only one pattern):

Person/object _____

Person/person _____

Object/object _____

Interaction pattern within the activity (check only one):

_____ *Intraindividual:* Action occurring within the mind or action involving the mind or a part of the body

- Requires no contact with another person or external object

_____ *Extraindividual:* Action directed by a person toward an object

- Requires no contact with another person

_____ *Aggregate:* Action directed by a person toward an object while in the company of other people who are also directing action toward an object

- Action is not directed toward each other

- No interaction between participants is needed

_____ *Interindividual:* Action of a competitive nature directed by one person toward another

_____ *Unilateral:* Action of a competitive nature among three or more people, one of whom is an antagonist or "it"

- Interaction is in simultaneous competitive relationship

_____ *Multilateral:* Action of a competitive nature among three or more people with no one person as an antagonist

_____ *Intragroup:* Action of a cooperative nature by two or more people intent on reaching a mutual goal

- Action requires positive verbal or nonverbal interaction

_____ *Intergroup:* Action of a competitive nature between two or more intragroups

Interaction with others

Physical contact:	1	2	3	4	5
	Little				Much

Competition:	1	2	3	4	5
	Little				Much

Emotional response:	1	2	3	4	5
	Little				Much

COGNITIVE IMPAIRMENT ASPECTS

(Check one or more where appropriate.)

_____ Mild cognitive impairment

_____ Moderate cognitive impairment

_____ Severe cognitive impairment

COGNITIVE ASPECTS

1. How many rules are there?

1	2	3	4	5
Few				Many

2. How complex are the rules?

1	2	3	4	5
Simple		Complex		

3. How much long-term memory is necessary?

1	2	3	4	5
Little			Much	

4. How much immediate recall is there?

1	2	3	4	5
Little			Much	

5. How much strategy does the activity require?

1   2   3   4   5

Little   Much

6. How much verbalization of thought process is required?

1   2   3   4   5

Little   Much

7. How much concentration is required?

1   2   3   4   5

Little   Much

AFFECTIVE ASPECTS

Circle the opportunities for the expression of the following emotions during this activity:

	Never				Often
Joy	**1**	**2**	**3**	**4**	**5**
Guilt	**1**	**2**	**3**	**4**	**5**
Pain	**1**	**2**	**3**	**4**	**5**
Anger	**1**	**2**	**3**	**4**	**5**
Fear	**1**	**2**	**3**	**4**	**5**
Frustration	**1**	**2**	**3**	**4**	**5**

SENSORIAL ASPECTS

What are the primary senses required for this activity?

Rate: 0 = not at all, 1 = rarely, 2 = occasionally, 3 = often

Touch _____

Taste _____

Sight _____

Hearing _____

Smell _____

ADMINISTRATIVE ASPECTS REGARDING THE THERAPIST

1. Leadership: Specific activity–skill response   _____

                             General activity–skill response   _____

                             Supervisory   _____

                             None needed   _____

2. Equipment: None required   _____

                             Specific commercial product   _____

                             Can be made   _____

3. Facilities: None required   _____

                             Specific natural environment   _____

                             Specific human-made environment   _____

4. Duration: Set time   _____

                             Natural end   _____

                             Continuous   _____

5. Participants: Any number   _____

                             Fixed number or multiple   _____

Sources for Art Supplies and Music

CREATIVE THINKING WHEN BRAINSTORMING PROJECTS

Look Around the Art Room

Often, when a therapist starts a new position in a facility, the only direction is toward a supply closet. More often than not, the closet has leftover supplies—some still usable, some that a therapist might not ever have used before. If the therapist is lucky, the supplies can suffice until his or her order is processed. A teaching exercise for therapy students is to have them bring to class four or five supplies that have no relation to each other and have them come up with as many projects for as many groups of clients as possible. The goal for students is to become acquainted with creative thinking, or what is commonly known as *thinking outside the box.*

Common Items and What to Do with Them

Old Clay   Clay easily can be made workable again by wetting a towel, twisting most of the water out of it, and wrapping it around the clay. Cover this with a plastic bag for a day or two, and the result will be workable clay and play dough. Play dough can be used on paper to create forms and shapes; this works well with individuals with communication problems.

Popsicle Sticks   The use of sticks can be very inexpensive yet very creative. Participants can make frames for artwork or photographs, bird houses, and flower sculptures.

Pipe Cleaners   Pipe cleaners now come in great colors and assorted sizes. They can be used to create bracelets and necklaces, as hair on clay animals, or in a group project in which everyone attaches his or her pipe cleaner to another person's, creating a huge string or chain. This is a safe and simple material to use.

Colored Paper   Colored paper is underrated; there are so many ways to stimulate participation with this basic art supply. Participants can trace their hand and cut it out or cut the paper into ribbon shapes to decorate activity rooms. Cut out leaves, hearts, pumpkins, fruits, and other objects and have participants color or write poems on them.

Tissue Paper   Paper comes in all sorts of shapes, such as human figures, flowers, squares, circles, and so forth. A popular project is to cover a bottle with tissue paper and then shellac it. Another good project is to make a stained glass look-alike by first creating a frame and then pasting together sheets of tissue paper; when held up to a window, it gives the illusion of stained glass.

Kitchen Supplies

Commonly, the kitchen in any facility has more supplies than the art closet. The following is a list of common objects that can have creative uses:

Paper plates

Plastic cups

Napkins

Coffee stirrers

Plastic trays

Empty cans from soup and coffee

Plastic bags for garbage

Nursing Supplies

Nursing departments are another creative place from which to get supplies. Be sure to get permission from the proper authority to use the following items so that the safety of residents is not compromised:

Plastic cups with lids

Containers that are no longer used

Plastic sterile gloves

Plastic liners

Plastic sticks

Look in the Garbage

The old saying, "One man's trash is another man's treasure," is actually creative thinking at work. Artwork can be made from scraps of metal, old lamp parts, sticks, and large cardboard that comes from carpet rolls, just to name a few. The following are only a few examples of commonly discarded things that make great project materials. Find out which day of the month the large garbage is collected, and watch what can be found!

Cardboard boxes

Cardboard rolls

Lampshades and parts

Used supplies

Bags of magazines

Bags of paper

What Can Be Found for Free

Yes, free! Many stores will save commonly discarded materials for a therapist; just ask! The following is a list of places from which a therapist can receive free materials; store owners, organizations, and so forth feel good that they are contributing to the program.

Fabric stores

Frame shops: pieces of colored paper and cardboard

Art suppliers: brushes, paints, strips of wood, cardboard

Flea markets: old toys, containers, buckets, hardware

Friends and family

Community: local women's club, garden club

Local colleges

What Can Be Found in Local Stores for Less Than $10.00

Paper plates

Paper cups

Balloons

Wood sticks

Straws

Plaster

Bowls

Wooden cigar boxes

Chinese take-out boxes

Where to Get Donations

Hardware stores

Cigarette shops

Department stores

Small town shops

Frame stores

Fabric shops

Drapery stores

BASIC START-UP MATERIALS NEEDED FOR A MUSIC AND MEDITATION PROGRAM (STEP 2)

You will need a tape player, CD player, portable media player, or digital audio player and music from the following six categories for a music and meditation program.

1. **Earth music**

   Albinoni: *Adagio for Strings and Organ*

   Giazotto, Conductor; Paillard Chamber Orchestra (RCA 654682-rc)

   Draws one into the inner world with pulling sounds; can affect the wakening of memories, yet tends to have a sad quality.

   Beethoven: *Symphony No. 7, Movement 2*

   Pablo Casals, Conductor; Marlboro Festival Orchestra, Sony Classical (SMK 45893)

   This piece often is described as music with a heartbeat. This music can awaken bodily responses or feelings that invite in-depth exploration.

   Vaughan Williams: *Pastoral Symphony*

   Bryden Thomson, Conductor; The London Symphony (CHAN 8594)

   This music has a sweeping effect and can be used to explore various moods; may evoke spiritual as well as emotional responses.

   Vaughan Williams: *Symphony No. 5*

   Andre Previn, Conductor; The London Symphony (RCA 605862RG)

The first three movements may be used in whole or in part to evoke a long (more than 30 minutes) inner journey. Evokes depth as it leads into varying moods. Overall, it is an uplifting piece of music.

2. Air music

Bach: *Orchestral Suite No. 3 in D Major, Movement 2*

Matthias Bamert, Conductor; BBC Philharmonic (CHAN 9259)

This is one of Bach's most famous pieces of music. It has an opening quality that stimulates imaging; it touches the soul.

Beethoven: *Symphony No. 9, Movement 1*

Eugene Ormandy, Conductor; Philadelphia Orchestra (CBS MYK 37241)

Exhilarating and vibrating sounds, this work can awaken creativity of all types. Excellent for renewing energy and rejuvenation.

Berlioz: *Symphonie Fantastique, Movement II*

Jean Martinon, Conductor; ORTF National Orchestra (EMI CZS762739-2)

This piece is described as celebratory; it is uplifting and moves into joyful sounds.

Ravel: *Introduction and Allegro*

Skaila Kanga and Academy of St. Martin-in-the-Fields, Chamber Ensemble (CHANDOS 8621)

3. Fire music

Bach: *Toccata and Fugue in D Minor*

Matthias Bamert, Conductor; BBC Philharmonic (CHAN 9259)

This piece evokes drama and power. Excellent to use for a drawing and painting program.

Brahms: *Symphony No. 3 in F Major, Opus 90, Movement 1*

George Szell, Conductor; Cleveland Orchestra (CBS MYK 37777)

This piece has been described as a large container in which one feels sweeping emotions.

Bruckner: *Symphony No. 8, Movement II: Scherzo*

Sir George Solti, Conductor; Chicago Symphony Orchestra (London 430 228)

Strong sounds that arouse instant feelings to surface in the mind.

Wagner: *Flying Dutchman, Overture* and *Tannhauser, Overture*

George Szell, Conductor; Cleveland Orchestra (CBS MYK 38486)

Flying Dutchman evokes excitement and passion and fires the imagination with images. *Tannhauser* has been described as having elements of earthy and spiritual sounds. Provides a depth and richness for individuals to experience and evokes a journey toward resolution of conflict.

4. Water music

Bartok: *Music for Strings, Percussion and Celesta, Movement 1: Andante Tranquillo*

Leonard Bernstein, Conductor; New York Philharmonic (CBS MK 42227)

Haunting music that has been described as possessing a universal quality to evoke a deep response.

Beethoven: *String Quartet in C Sharp Minor, Opus 131*

Alban Berg Quartet (EMI CDC7 47137-2)

This music has been described as having a nurturing quality. It is smooth and can bring attention to the inner child.

Brahms: *Symphony No. 2, Movement III, Andante*

George Szell, Conductor; Cleveland Orchestra (CBS MYK 337258)

This piece is uplifting and lively; it has the ability to evoke positive inner responses.

Brahms: *Symphony No. 3, Movements II and III*

This music is inspiring and uplifting and can be used to stimulate imagery.

5. Descent music

Bach: *Come Sweet Death* and *Prelude in B Minor*

Matthias Bamert, Conductor; BBC Philharmonic (CHAN 9259)

Come Sweet Death evokes feelings of sadness. *Prelude in B Minor* is string music that has tension within the sounds. It has a deep, probing effect, so be careful when using it, because of its strong ability to stir emotions.

Beethoven: *Symphony No. 3 "Eroica," Movement 2*

Sir Neville Marriner, Conductor; Academy of St. Martin-in-the-Fields (Phillips 410 044)

This piece has a slow and somber effect, which can be used in a grieving situation.

Holst: *The Planets, Saturn*

Gyorgy Ligeti, Conductor; Boston Symphony (Stereo 419 475-2)

Excellent piece for deep exploration. This piece pulls you into deep subconscious issues yet resonates with hope and resolution.

6. **Ascent music**

Bach: *Mass in B Minor, "Qui Tollis"*

Karl Richer, Conductor; Munich Bach Choir and Orchestra (Musikfest 413 688-2)

This piece has been described as inspirational, with awe and reverence.

Mahler: *Symphony No. 5, Movement III*

Sir John Barbirolli, Conductor; New Philharmonia Orchestra (EMI CDM7 69186-2)

This piece features the harp and has a true spirit of transcendence.

Mozart: *Vesperae Solennes, Laudate Dominum*

Joseph Silverstein, Conductor; Utah Symphony Orchestra with Frederica von Stade and the Mormon Tabernacle Choir (London 436 284-2)

Lifts one to inspirational heights. This piece has singing and orchestration.

BASIC START-UP MATERIALS NEEDED FOR A DRAWING AND PAINTING PROGRAM (STEP 3)

11" × 14" paper or 18" × 24" pads of white paper

11" × 14" paper or 18" × 24" pads of lower-grade paper

Pastel chalks

Colored pencils

Colored markers with various tip sizes and widths

Oil crayons/pastels

Drawing pencils: HB, 2B, 3B, 6B (numbers indicate hardness of lead)

Erasers

Watercolors

Watercolor brushes (several sizes)

Plastic trays for mixing and holding water

Set of acrylic paints, brushes, disposable palettes, and canvases

Scissors

White school-grade paper glue

Glue sticks

Colored glitter or sand

BASIC START-UP MATERIALS NEEDED FOR A SCULPTURE PROGRAM (STEP 4)

Crayola Model Magic: tubs of white, red, yellow, and blue

Omya air-dry clay

Modeling tools

Rolling pins

Clay hammers/various surfaces

Clay cutters

Clay extruding gun

Crayola fun shapes on rolling pins

Fimo (plain) & Fimo mixed color kit

Push molds

Character molds: hands, feet, heads

Sculpey modeling clay

Rigid Wrap (nontoxic wrap that contains plaster; easily molded onto all types of surfaces)

Fiberboard cones

Celluclay instant papier-mâché

Armature wire netting

Paris craft (used over wire)

Plaster of Paris

Plaster of Paris molds

Graphic Organizing Tools

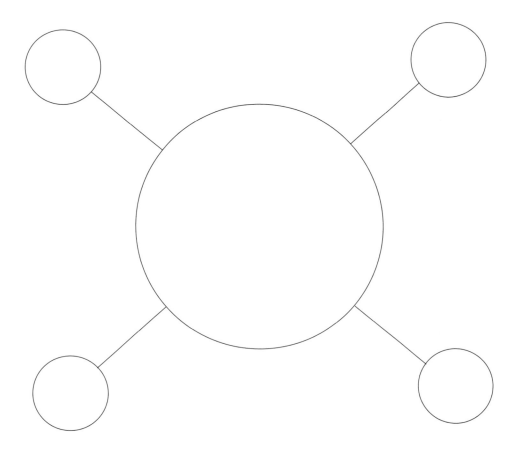

Descriptive patterns can be used to organize facts or characteristics about specific people, places, things, and events. This is the simplest form of graphic display. Each participant receives a copy to start working on a particular theme. If the chosen theme is holidays, for example, then each participant can write down the most significant four holidays that they remember. Then the therapist can display on the group chart the four most common among the group. There are many possibilities for how the group can proceed to pick one holiday to use as the theme.

Another example of how this descriptive pattern chart can be used is by starting the group with music. The therapist can play a tape of nature sounds and then have a theme discussion regarding the sounds heard. Each individual can be asked to share a thought that came to mind while listening to the nature sounds. This enables each individual to describe a personal memory regarding a special moment or an event.

PROCESS AND CAUSATION PATTERNS

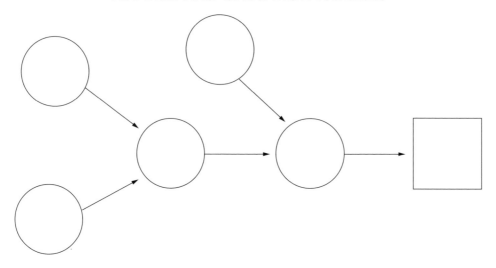

Process and causation patterns can organize information into a causal network that leads to a specific outcome or into a sequence of steps that lead to a specific product, idea, or elements of a theme. If the group has chosen making flowers as a theme for an art activity, then a process/causation chart can be used to organize the many different ways in which a flower can be made. For example, a flower can be made individually, then organized into a bunch, and then placed into an arrangement. If a therapist is working with a cognitively challenged group, then this process is crucial for visually organizing thoughts and thereby preventing frustration and anxiety.

GENERALIZATION PATTERNS

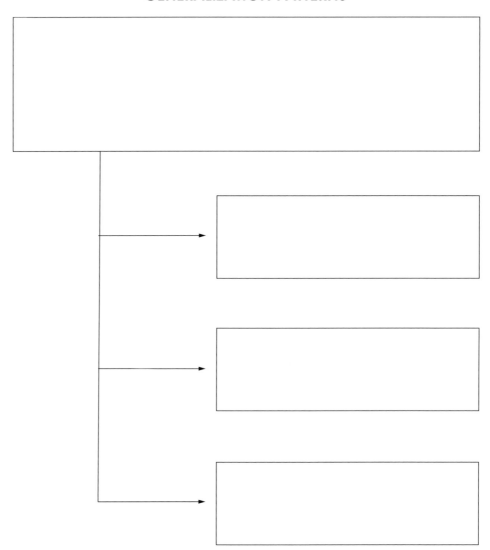

Generalization patterns organize information into generalized supporting information. This is a good diagram to use to back up theme information. This graphic organizer could be used to give examples of various cars that the clients owned or of types of trees that grow in various states.

SEQUENCE PATTERNS

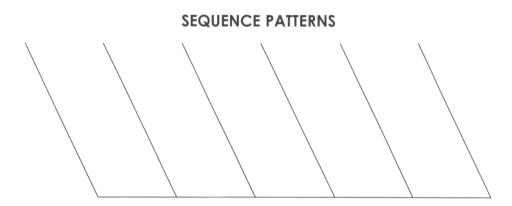

Sequence patterns organize events in a specific chronological order. If you were discussing events in history chronologically, then this would be an excellent graphic organizer. This also is an excellent cognitive tool to stimulate recall abilities.

PROBLEM-SOLVING PATTERNS

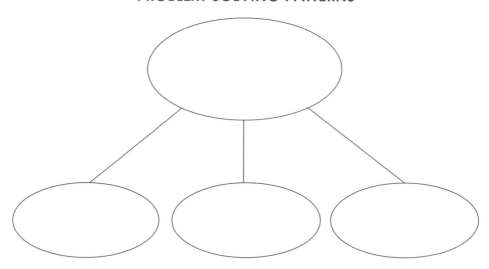

Problem-solving patterns organize information into an identified problem and its possible solutions. This is another excellent format for dealing with conflict or problems. It gives the user direction in the narrative, and it gives the participants the ability to interact and be heard. A good example of problem solving is when two people who live together cannot adjust to the living environment. This technique can enable clients to work out living arrangements by identifying what is personally important to each one individually.

CONCEPT PATTERNS

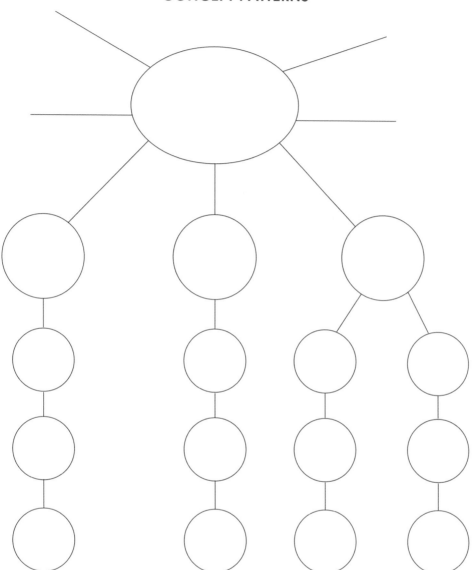

Concept patterns are the most general of all patterns. Like descriptive patterns, they deal with people, places, things, and events, but they represent an entire class or category and usually illustrate specific examples and defining characteristics of the concept. An example of using a concept pattern is to define a special evening event and all of the various foods needed.

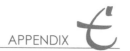

Themes in the TTAP Method

The following themes have been developed successfully into theme programming.

changes	angels	food
symbols	life lessons	flowers
seasons	summer	family
culture	smells	jobs
systems	textures	religion
facts	fashion	holidays
communication	movies	music
languages	personalities	dances
body language	games	nations
colors	months	current events
animals	decades	women's issues
the ocean	centuries	men's issues
inventions	families	hobbies
fantasy	children	the arts
conflict	memories	the sciences
solutions	travel	the humanities
traditions	mysteries	
mountains	books	

References

Aadlandsvik, R. (2007). Education, poetry, and the process of growing old. *Educational Gerontology, 33*(8), 665–678.

Abrisqueta-Gomez, J., Brucki, S., Canali, F., Oliveira, E., Ponce, C., Vieira, V., & Bueno, O. (2002). Neuropsychological rehabilitation program in cognitive impairment and dementia. In L. Battistin, M. Dam, & P. Tonin (Eds). *Proceedings of the 3rd World Congress Neurological Rehabilitation* (pp. 399–407). Venice: Monduzzi Editore.

Abrisqueta-Gomez, J., Canali, F., Vieira, V., Aguiar, A., Ponce, C., Brucki, S., & Bueno, O. (2004). A longitudinal study of a neuropsychological rehabilitation program in Alzheimer's disease. *Archives of Neuro-Psychiatry,62*(3), 778–783.

Acevedo, A., & Loewenstein, D. (2007). Nonpharmacological cognitive interventions in aging and dementia. *Journal of Geriatric Psychiatry and Neurology, 20*(4), 239–249.

Adams, T. (2008). Kitwood's approach to dementia and dementia care: A critical but appreciative review. *Journal of Advanced Nursing, 23*(5), 948–953.

Addis, D.R., Wong, A.T., & Schacter, D.L. (2008). Age-related changes in the episodic simulation of future events. *Psychological Science, 19*(1), 33–41.

Alders, A., & Levine-Madori, L. (2010). The effect of art therapy on cognitive performance of Hispanic/Latino older adults. *Art Therapy: Journal of the American Art Therapy Association, 27*(3), 127–135.

Aldridge, D. (2000). It's not what you do but the way that you do it. In D. Aldridge (Ed.), *Music therapy in dementia care* (pp. 9–32). London: Jessica Kingsley Publishers.

Alzheimer's Association. (2011). 2011 Alzheimer's disease facts and figures. *Alzheimer's & Dementia, 7*(2).

American Art Therapy Association. (2007). *AATA governmental affairs 2006–2007 sourcebook*. Available at www.arttherapy.org/upload/file/GACsourcebook2006_07.pdf

American Health Assistance Foundation. (2009). *Brain with Alzheimer's disease.* Available at http://www.ahaf.org/alzheimers/about/understanding/brain-with-alzheimers.html

American Psychiatric Association. (2000). *Diagnostic and statistical manual of mental disorders* (4th ed. rev.). Arlington, VA: American Psychiatric Association.

American Therapeutic Recreation Association. (2008). *Dementia practice guideline for recreational therapy: Treatment of disturbing behaviors.* Hattiesburg, MS: American Therapeutic Recreation Association.

Anderson, A.J. (2002). Treatment of depression in older adults. *International Journal of Psychosocial Rehabilitation, 6,* 69–78.

Anderson, W., & Krathwohl, R. (Eds.). (2000). *A taxonomy for learning, teaching and assessing: A revision of Bloom's Taxonomy of educational objectives.* New York: Longman.

Anderson, W., & Sosniak, A. (Eds.). (1994). *Bloom's taxonomy: A forty-year retrospective.* Chicago, IL: University of Chicago Press.

Arehart-Treichel, J. (2001). Scientists identify brain area first affected by Alzheimer's. *Psychiatric News, 36*(20), 23.

Avila, R., Bottino, C., Carvalho, I., Santos, C., Seral, C., & Miotto, E. (2004). Neuropsychological rehabilitation of memory deficits and activities of daily living in patients with Alzheimer's disease: A pilot study. *Brazilian Journal of Medical and Biological Research, 37*(11), 1721–1729.

Baltes, P.M., Reese, H.W., & Lipsitt, L. (1980). Life-span developmental psychology. *Annual Review of Psychology, 31,* 65–110.

Barrett, C.E. (1986). In search of brain–behavior relationships in dementia and the Lauria-Nebraska neuropsychology battery. In E.D. Taira (Ed.), *Physical and occupational therapy in geriatrics: Current trends in geriatric rehabilitation* (pp. 113–139). New York: Haworth Press.

Bayles, A., Tomoeda, C. & Trosset, M. (1992). Relation of linguistic communication abilities of Alzheimer's patients to stage of disease. *Journal of Brain and Language, 42*(4), 454–472.

Bell, V., & Troxel, D. (1997). *The Best Friends approach to Alzheimer's care.* Baltimore, MD: Health Professions Press.

Beurs, E., Beekman, A., Van Balkom, A., Deeg, D., Van Dyck, R., & Van Tilbug, W. (1999). Consequences of anxiety in older persons: Its effect on disability, well-being and use of health services. *Psychological Medicine, 29*(3), 583–593

Blacker, D., Lee, H., Muzikansky, A., Martin, E., Tanzi, R., McArdle, J., Moss, M., & Albert, M. (2007). Neuropsychological measures in normal individuals that predict subsequent cognitive decline. *Archives of Neurology, 64*(6), 862–871.

Blatner, A. (2003). Using creativity to explore in psychotherapy. *Psychiatric Times, 20* (6). Available at, http://www.psychiatrictimes.com/display/article/10168/48321

Bloom, S., & Krathwohl, D. (1956). *Taxonomy of educational objectives: The classification of educational goals, by a committee of college and university examiners.* New York: Longmans.

Bohlmeijer, E., Smit, F., & Cuijpers, P. (2003). Effects of reminiscence and life review on late-life depression: A meta-analysis. *International Journal of Geriatric Psychiatry, 18,* 1088–1094.

Boise, L., & White, D. (2004). The family's role in person-centered care: Practice considerations. *Journal of Psychosocial Nursing and Mental Health Services, 42*(5), 12–20.

Bohlmeijer, F., Valenkamp, M., Westerhof, G., Smi, F., & Cuijpers, P. (2005). Creative reminiscence as an early intervention for depression: Results of a pilot project. *Aging & Mental Health, 9*(4), 302–304.

Bookheimer, S., Magdalena, H., Strojwas, B., Cohen, M., Saunders, A., Pericak-Vance, M., Mazziotta, J., & Small, G. (2000). Patterns of brain activation in people at risk for Alzheimer's disease. *New England Journal of Medicine, 343*(7), 450–456.

Bossen, A., Specht, J., & McKenzie, E. (2009). Needs of people with early-stage Alzheimer's disease: Reviewing the evidence. *Journal of Gerontological Nursing, 35*(3), 8–15.

Boston University. (2009, May 1). Mild Alzheimer's: Photos more useful than words. *ScienceDaily.* Available at http://www.sciencedaily.com/releases/2009/04/090430111637.htm

Bottino, C., Carvalho, I., Alvarez, A. (2002). Cognitive rehabilitation in Alzheimer's disease patients: Multidisciplinary team report. *Archives of Neuropsychiatry, 60,* 70–79.

Bourgeois, M., Dijkstra, K., Burgio, L., & Allen-Burge, R. (2001). Memory aids as an augmentative and alternative communication strategy for nursing home residents with dementia. *Augmentative and Alternative Communication, 17*(3), 196–210.

Boylin, W., Gordon, S., & Nehrke, M. (1976). Reminiscence and ego integrity in institutionalized elderly. *Gerontologist, 16,* 118–124.

Braak, H., & Braak, E. (1997). Frequency of stages of Alzheimer's-related lesions in different age categories. *Neurobiology of Aging, 18,* 351–357.

Breitbart, W., Gibson, C., Poppito, S. R., & Berg, A. (2004). Psychotherapeutic interventions at the end of life: A focus on meaning and spirituality. *Canadian Journal of Psychiatry, 49*(6), 366–372.

Brierley, E., Guthrie, E., Busby, C., Marino-Francis, F., Byrne, J., & Burns, A. (2003). Psychodynamic interpersonal therapy for early Alzheimer's disease. *British Journal of Psychotherapy, 19*(4), 435–446.

Broadbent, E., Cooper, F., FitzGerald, P., & Parkes, R. (1982). The Cognitive Failures Questionnaire (CFQ) and its correlates. *British Journal of Clinical Psychology, 21,* 1–16.

Brodaty, H., & Moore, M. (1997). The clock drawing test for dementia of the Alzheimer's type: A comparison of three scoring methods from a memory disorders clinic. *International Journal of Geriatric Psychiatry, 12,* 619–627.

Brooker, D. (2004). What is person-centred care in dementia? *Reviews in Clinical Gerontology, 13,* 215–222.

Brookmeyer, R., Corrada, M., Curriero, F., & Kawas, C. (2002). Survival following a diagnosis of Alzheimer disease. *Archives of Neurology, 59,* 1764–1767.

Brookmeyer, R., Gray, S., & Kawas, C. (1998). Projections of Alzheimer's disease in the United States and the public health impact of delaying disease onset. *American Journal of Public Health, 88*(9), 1337–1342.

Brotons, M. (2000). An overview of the music therapy literature relating to elderly people. In D. Aldridge (Ed.), *Music therapy in dementia care* (pp. 33–62). London: Jessica Kingsley Publishers.

Brotons, M., & Marti, P. (2003, Summer). Music therapy with Alzheimer's patients and their family caregivers: A pilot project. *Journal of Music Therapy, 40*(2), 138–150.

Brown, J. W. (1999). Neuropsychology and the self-concept. *Journal of Nervous & Mental Disease, 187*(3), 131–141.

Bruscia, K., & Grocke, D. (2002). *Guided imagery and music: The Bonny Method and beyond.* Gilsum, NH: Barcelona Publishers.

Buckwalter, K., Burgener, S., & Buettner, L. (2009) Review of exemplar programs for persons in early stage Alzheimer's disease. *Journal of Gerontological*

Nursing Research, 1(4). Available at http://www.geronurseresearch.com/view. asp?rID=32166

Buettner, L. (1988). Utilizing developmental theory and adaptive equipment with regressed geriatric patients in therapeutic recreation. *Therapeutic Recreation Journal, 22*(3), 72–79.

Buettner, L. (1999, July). Simple pleasures: A multilevel, sensorimotor intervention for nursing home residents with dementia. *American Journal of Alzheimer's Disease,* 41–52.

Buettner, L. (2006). Peace of mind: A pilot community based program for older adults with memory loss. *American Journal of Recreation Therapy, 5*(1), 42–48.

Buettner, L., & Ferrario, C. (1998). Therapeutic recreation and nursing: A team intervention for nursing home residents with dementia. *Annual in Therapeutic Recreation, 7,* 15–26.

Buettner, L., & Kolanowski, A. (2003). Practice guidelines for recreation therapy in the care of people with dementia (CE). *Geriatric Nursing, 24*(1), 18–25.

Bugental, J. The third force in psychology. *Journal of Humanistic Psychology, (4)*1, 19–25.

Burgener, C., & Dickson-Putman, J. (1999). Assessing patients in the early stages of irreversible dementia: Relevance of patient perspectives. *Journal of Gerontological Nursing, 25*(2), 33–41.

Burgener, C., Buettner, L., Beattie, E., & Rose, K. (2009). Effectiveness of community-based, nonpharmacological interventions for early-stage dementia: conclusions and recommendations. *Journal of Gerontology Nursing, 35*(3), 50–57.

Burgener, C., Gilbert, R., & Mathy, R., (2007). The effects of a multi-modal intervention on cognitive, physical, and affective outcomes of persons with early stage dementia. *Journal of Alzheimer's Disease and Related Disorders, 12,* 143–156.

Burke, S., & Barnes, A. (2006). Neural plasticity in the ageing brain. *Nature Reviews of Neuroscience, 7,* 30–40. Available at doi:10.1038/nrn1809.

Butler, R. (1963). The life review: An interpretation of reminiscence in the aged. *Psychiatry, 26,* 65–76.

Butters, M.A., Becker, J. T., Nebes, R.D., Zmuda, M.D., Mulsant, B.H., & Pollock, B.G. (2000). Changes in cognitive functioning following treatment of late-life depression. *American Journal of Psychiatry, 157,* 1949–1954.

Camp, C.J. (1989). Facilitation of new learning in Alzheimer's disease. In C. Gilmore, P.J. Whitehouse, & M.L. Wykle (Eds.), *Memory aging and dementia: Theory, assessment and treatment* (pp. 212–225). New York: Springer.

Cappeliez, P., O'Rourke, N. & Chaudhury, H. (2005). Functions of reminiscence and mental health in later life. *Aging & Mental Health, 9*(4), 295–301.

Carver, C.S. (2004). Negative affects deriving from the behavioural approach system. *Emotion, 4,* 3–22.

Cash, A. (2006). Music for hysterectomy and Alzheimer's patients. Available at http://healingmusicenterprises.com/ezine/2006-07.html#Alzheimer%20 Patients%20Music

Center for Medicare and Medicaid Services. (2009, January 27). MDS 3.0 for Nursing Homes. Available at http://www.cms.hhs.gov/NursingHomeQuality Inits/25_NHQIMDS30.asp

Centers for Disease Control and Prevention. (2009). Deaths: Preliminary data for 2009. *National Vital Statistics Report, 59*(4). Available at http://www.cdc.gov/ nchs/products/nvsr.htm#vol60

Chapman, B., Duberstein, P., & Lyness, J. (2007). Personality traits, education, and health-related quality of life among older adult primary care patients. *Journals of Gerontology. Series B: Psychological Sciences and Social Sciences, 62*(6), P343–352.

Chertkow, H., Verret, L. Bergmen, H., et al. (2001). Predicting progression to dementia in elderly subjects with mild cognitive impairment: A multidisciplinary approach. Contemporary Clinical Issues. Plenary Session, 53rd Annual Meeting of the American Academy of Neurology, Philadelphia.

Clare, L., Pistrang, N., & Pearce, A. (2002). Managing sense of self. *Dementia, 1*(2), 173–192.

Clare, L., Wilson, B., Carter, G., Roth, I., & Hodges, J. (2004). Awareness in early-stage dementia: Relationship to outcome of cognitive rehabilitation intervention. *Journal of Clinical and Experimental Neuropsychology, 26*(2), 215–226.

Coblentz, J.M., Mattis, S., Zingesser, L.H., Kasoff, S.S., Wisniewski, H.M., & Katzman, R. (1973). Presenile dementia: Clinical evaluation of cerebrospinal fluid dynamics. *Archives of Neurology, 29,* 299–308.

Coghill, R. (2000). *Exploring the nervous system: Brain imaging.* Available at http://Faculty.Washington.edu/chudler/image.html

Cohen, G. (2006). *The mature mind: The positive power of the aging brain.* New York: Basic Books.

Cotrell, V., & Schulty, R. (1993). The perspective of the patient with Alzheimer's disease: A neglected dimension of dementia research. *Gerontologist, 33,* 205–211.

Council of Europe/European Commission. (2002). Training in action. In *Training Essentials (T-Kit No. 6)* (pp. 81–92). Available at http://www.salto-youth.net/tools/toolbox/tool/training-kit-on-training-essentials-t-kit-series.71/

Craig, S.D., Graesser, A.C., Sullins, J., & Gholson, B. (2004). Affect and learning: An exploratory look into the role of affect in learning with AutoTutor. *Journal of Educational Media, 29,* 241–250.

Crits-Cristoph, P., Demorest, A., Muenz, L. R., & Baranackie, K. (1994). Consistency of interpersonal themes for patients in psychotherapy. *Journal of Personality, 62*(4), 499–526.

Csikszentmihalyi, M. (1991). *Flow: The psychology of optimal experience.* New York: Harper and Row.

Csikszentmihalyi, M. (1997). *Finding flow: The psychology of engagement with everyday life.* New York: Basic Books.

Cummins, P., Giordano, J., Lewis, J., Peruyera, G., & Siegel, J. (2008). *Recreational therapy in the nursing home.* American Therapeutic Recreation Association.

Curtis, M.A., Penney, E.B., Pearson, A.G., van Roon-Mom, W. M.C., Butterworth, N.J., Dragunow, M., Connor, B., & Faull, R. (2003). Increased cell proliferation and neurogenesis in the adult human Huntington's disease brain. *Proceedings of the National Academy of Sciences, 100*(15), 9023–9027.

Damasio, A.R. (2003). *Looking for Spinoza: Joy, sorrow, and the feeling brain.* Orlando, FL: Harcourt.

Davie, J.E., Azuma, T., Goldinger, S.D., Connor, D.J., Sabbagh, M.N., & Silverberg, N.B. (2004). Sensitivity to expectancy violations in healthy aging and mild cognitive impairment. *Neuropsychology, 18*(2), 269–275.

Deci, E.L., & Ryan, R.M. (2002). The paradox of achievement: The harder you push, the worse it gets. In J. Aronson (Ed.), *Improving academic achievement: Impact of psychological factors on education* (pp. 61–87). Orlando, FL: Academic Press.

de Leon, M., Convit, A., Wolf, O.T., Tarshish, C.Y., DeSanti, S., Rusinek, H., et al. (2001). Prediction of cognitive decline in normal elderly subjects with 2-[^{18}F]fluoro-2-deoxy-d-glucose/positron-emission tomography (FDG/PET). *Proceedings of the National Academy of Sciences, 98*(19), 10966–10971.

De Petrillo, L., & Winner, E. (2005). Does art improve mood? A test of a key assumption underlying art therapy. *Art Therapy, 22,* 205–212.

Diamond, K. (2000). *Older brains and new connections.* San Luis Obispo, CA: Davidson Publications.

Dirkx, J. (2001). The power of feelings: Emotion, imagination, and the construction of meaning in adult learning. *New Directions for Adult and Continuing Education, 89,* 63–72.

Dombeck, M. (1983). The theme-centered interactional group model in professional education. *Small Group Research, 14*(3), 275–300.

Dunne, T., Neargarder, S., Cipolloni, P., & Cronin-Golomb, A. (2004). Visual contrast enhances food and liquid intake in advanced Alzheimer's disease. *Clinical Nutrition, 23*(4), 533–538.

Dweck, C.S. (2002). Messages that motivate: How praise molds students' beliefs, motivation, and performance (in surprising ways). In J. Aronso (Ed.), *Improving academic achievement: Impact of psychological factors on education* (pp. 61–87). Orlando, FL: Academic Press.

Eaton, L.G., Doherty, K.L. & Widrick, R.M. (2007). A review of research and methods used to establish art therapy as an effective treatment method for traumatized children. *Arts in Psychotherapy, 34,* 256–262.

Erikson, E.H. (1963). *Childhood and society* (2nd ed.). New York: W. W. Norton.

Erikson, E.H., Erikson, J.M., & Kivnick, H.Q. (1986). *Vital involvement in old age.* New York: W. W. Norton.

Eslinger, P., & Damasio, A. (1986). Preserved motor learning in Alzheimer's disease: Implications for anatomy and behavior. *Journal of Neuroscience, 6,* 3006–3009.

Fernandez-Ballesteros, R., Zamarron, M.D., Tarraga, L., Moya, R., & Iniguez, J. (2003). Cognitive plasticity in healthy, mild cognitive impairment (MCI) subjects and Alzheimer's disease patients: A research project in Spain. *European Psychologist, 8*(3), 148–159.

Fillenbaum, G., Heyman, A., Williams, K., Prosnit, B., & Burchett, B. (1990). Sensitivity and specificity of standard screens for cognitive impairment and dementia among elderly Black and White community residents. *Journal of Clinical Epidemiology, 43,* 651–660.

Finnemore, G. (2009). *Brain fitness and training heads towards its tipping point.* Available at http://www.sharpbrains.com/blog/2009/01/19/brain-fitnesstraining-heads-towards-its-tipping-point

Fiore, J., Becker, J., & Coppel, D.B. (1983). Social network interactions: A buffer or a stress? *American Journal of Community Psychology, 11*(2), 423–439.

Flood, M., and Phillips, K. (2007). Creativity in older adults: A plethora of possibilities. *Mental Health Nursing, 28*(4), 389–411.

Folstein, F., Folstein, E., & McHugh P. (1975). Mini-Mental State: A practical method for grading the cognitive state of patients for the clinician. *Journal of Psychiatry Research, 12,* 189–198.

Fratiglioni, L, Paillard-Borg, S., & Winblad, B. (2004). An active and socially integrated lifestyle in late life might protect against dementia. *Lancet Neurology Journal, 3,* 343–353.

Frazer, J., Christensen, H., & Griffiths, M. (2005). Effectiveness of treatments for depression in older people. *Medical Journal of Australia, 182*(12), 627–632.

Garand, L., Buckwalter, K., & Hall, G. (2000). The biological basis of behavioral symptoms in dementia. *Issues in Mental Health Nursing, 21*(1), 91–107.

Gardner, H. (1982). *Art, mind, and brain.* New York: Basic Books.

Gardner, H. (1997). *Extraordinary minds: Portraits of exceptional individuals and an examination of our extraordinariness.* New York: Basic Books.

Gault, G. M. (2008). Neurodevelopmental theory: NDT treatment for the person with a neurological injury. Available at http://ezinearticles.com/?Neurode velopmental-Theory-NDT-Treatment-For-The-Person-With-A-Neurological-Injury

Gawain, S. (1996). *Creative visualization meditations.* Novato, CA: New World Library.

Gerdner, L. (2000). Effects of individualized versus classical "relaxation" music on the frequency of agitation in elderly persons with Alzheimer's disease and related disorders. *International Psychogeriatrics, 12,* 49–65.

Gilhooly, M., Zarit, S., & Berrin, J. (1986). *The dementia's: Policy and management.* Englewood Cliffs, NJ: Prentice Hall.

Gilley, W., Wilson, L., Bienias, L., Bennett, A., & Evans, A. (2004). Predictors of depression symptoms in persons with Alzheimer's disease. *Journal of Gerontology: Psychological Sciences, 59*(2), 75–83.

Golomb, J., Kluger, A., & Ferris, S. (2002). *Evidence-based dementia practice.* Oxford, England: Oxford University Press.

Golomb, J., Kluger, A., de Leon, M. J., Ferris, S., Mittelman, M., Cohen, J., & George, A. E. (1996). Hippocampal formation size predicts declining memory performance in normal aging. *Neurology, 47,* 810–813.

Gordon, M. (1972). *Theme-centered interaction: An original focus on counseling and education.* Washington, DC: National Educational Press.

Gray, J., Braver, T., & Raichle, M. (2002). Integration of emotion and cognition in the lateral prefrontal cortex. *Proceedings of the National Academy of Science, 99*(6), 4115–4120.

Green, K.N., Billings, L.M., McGaugh, J.L., & LaFerla, F.M. (2007). Learning decreases Ab56, tau pathology, and ameliorates behavioral decline in 3xTg-AD mice. *Journal of Neuroscience, 27*(4): 751–761.

Grober, E., Dickson, D., & Sliwinski, M.J. (1999). Memory and mental status correlates of modified Braak staging. *Neurobiology of Aging, 20,* 573–579.

Grobstein, P. (2007). Interdisciplinarity, transdisciplinarity, and beyond: The brain, story sharing, and social organization. *Journal of Research Practice, 3*(2), M21.

Grobstein, P. (2008). The brain as a learner/inquirer/creator: Some implications of its organization for individual and social well-being. Available at http://serendip.brynmawr.edu/exchange/grobstein/olympiad07

Gurland, B., Wilder, D., Lantigua, R., Stern, Y., Chen, J. (1999). Rates of dementia in three ethno-racial groups. *International Journal of Geriatric Psychiatry, 14*(6), 481–493.

Haight, B. (2007). *The handbook of structured life review.* Baltimore: Health Professions Press.

Haight, K., & Burnside, I. (1993). Reminiscence and life review: Explaining the differences. *Archives of Psychiatric Nursing, 7,* 91–98.

Haight, K., Bachman, L., Hendrix, S., Wagner, T., Meeks, A., & Johnson, J. (2003). Life review: Treating the dyadic family unit with dementia. *Clinical Psychology & Psychotherapy, 10*(3), 165–174.

Hall, J., Thomas, K., & Everitt, B. (2000). Rapid and selective induction of BDNF expression in the hippocampus during contextual learning. *Nature Neuroscience, 3*, 533–535.

Hamann, S. (2001). Cognitive and neural mechanisms of emotional memory. *TRENDS in Cognitive Sciences, 5*(9), 394–400.

Hass-Cohen, N., & Carr, R. (Eds.). (2008). *Art therapy and clinical neuroscience.* London: Jessica Kingsley.

Hebert, L., Wilson R., Gilley, D., Beckett L., Scherr, P., Bennett, D., & Evans, D. (2000). Decline of language among women and men with Alzheimer's disease. *Journals of Gerontology Series B: Psychological Sciences and Social Sciences, 55*, 354–361.

Hebert, L., Beckett, L., Scherr, P., Evans, D. (2001). Annual incidence of Alzheimer disease in the United States projected to the years 2000 through 2050. *Alzheimer Disease and Associated Disorders: An International Journal, 15*(4), 169–173.

Hehman, J., German, T., & Klein, S. (2005). Impaired self-recognition from recent photographs in a case of late–stage Alzheimer's disease. *Autobiographical Memory: Empirical Applications, 23*(1), 118–124.

Henri, M., & Cattin, D. (2005). *The human hippocampus: Functional anatomy, vascularization, and serial sections with MRI.* New York: Springer.

Hornecker, E. (2001). Process and structure: Dialectics instead of dichotomies. Position paper for E-CSCW Workshop on Structure and Process: The Interplay of Routine and Informed Action. Bonn, September 2001.

Hughes, C.P., Berg, L., Danziger, W.L., Cohen, L.A., & Martin, R.L. (1982). A new clinical scale for the staging of dementia. *British Journal of Psychiatry, 140*, 566–572.

Ishii, T. (2004). Distribution of Alzheimer's neurofibrillary changes in the brain stem and hypothalamus of senile dementia. *Acta Neuropathologica, 6*(2). Available at http://www.springerlink.com/content/l30q85h773302547/

Jarrott, S. (2003). Intergenerational activities involving persons with dementia: An observational assessment. *American Journal of Alzheimer's Disease and Other Dementias, 18*(1), 31–37.

Jeff A., Small, J., Gutman, G., Makela, S., & Hillhouse, B. (2003). Effectiveness of communication strategies used by caregivers of persons with Alzheimer's disease during activities of daily living. *Journal of Speech, Language, and Hearing Research, 46*, 353–367.

Johnson, C. (2000). Therapeutic recreation treats depression in the elderly. *Home Health Care Services Quarterly, 18*(2), 79–90.

Jonas-Simpson, C., & Mitchell, G. (2005). Giving voice to expressions of quality of life for persons living with dementia through story, music, and art. *Alzheimer's Care Quarterly, 6*(1), 52–61.

Jung, C.G. (1963). *Collected works of C.G. Jung: mysterium coniunctionis: An inquiry into the separation and synthesis of psychic opposites in alchemy.* New York: Routledge.

Kane, R., & Kane, R.L. (1981). *Assessing the elderly. A practical guide to measurement.* Lexington, MA: Lexington Books.

Kaplan, F. (2000). *Art, science and art therapy*. Philadelphia: Jessica Kingsley.

Kasl-Godley, J., & Gatz, M. (2000). Psychosocial intervention for individuals with dementia: An integration of theory, therapy, and a clinical understanding of dementia. *Clinical Psychology Review, 20*, 755–782.

Kensinger, E., Brierley, B., Medford, N., Growdon, J., & Corkin, S. (2002). The effects of normal aging and Alzheimer's disease on emotional memory. *Emotion, 2*(2), 118–134.

Kinsella, G., Mullaly, E., Rand, E., Ong, B., Burton, C., Price, S., Phillips, M., & Storey, E. (2008). Early intervention for mild cognitive impairment: A randomized controlled trial. *Journal of Neurology, Neurosurgery & Psychiatry*. Available at http://jnnp.bmj.com/cgi/rapidpdf/jnnp.2008.148346v1

Klee, T. (1990). Object relations theory. *American Journal of Psychiatry, 147*(7), 961–962.

Kluger, A., Ferris, S.H., Golomb, J., Mittelman, M., & Reisberg, B. (1999). Neuropsychological prediction of decline to dementia in nondemented elderly. *Journal of Geriatric Psychiatry and Neurology, 12*, 168–179.

Kontos, P. (2005). Embodied selfhood in Alzheimer's disease. *Dementia, 4*(4), 553–570.

Kort, B., Reilly, R., & Picard, R. (2001). An affective model of interplay between emotions and learning: Reengineering educational pedagogy-building: A learning companion. In *Advanced Learning Technologies, 2001. Proceedings of the IEEE International Conference* (pp. 43–46).

Kramer, E. (2000). *Art as therapy*. London, England: Jessica Kinglsey.

Kramer, A.F., Bherer, L., Colcombe, S. J., Dong, W., & Greenough, W.T. (2004). Environmental influences on cognitive and brain plasticity during aging. *Journal of Gerontology: Medical Science, 59*(9), 940–957.

Kuhn, D., Ortigara, A., & Kasayka, R. (2000). Dementia care mapping: An innovative tool to measure person-centered care. *Alzheimer's Care Quarterly, 1*(3), 7–15.

Kumara, R., Dearb, K., Christensenb, H., Ilschnerb, S., Meslinb, S., & Sachdevc, P. (2005). Prevalence of mild cognitive impairment in 60- to 64-year-old community-dwelling individuals: The Personality and Total Health through Life 60+ Study. *Dementia and Geriatric Cognitive Disorders, 19*, 67–74.

Kuwahara, N., Shinji, A., Yasuda, K., & Kuwabara, K. (2006). Networked reminiscence therapy for individuals with dementia by using photo and video sharing. In *Proceedings of the 8th International ACM SIGACCESS Conference on Computers and Accessibility*. Available at http://portal.acm.org/citation.cfm?id=1169010

Landerman, R., George, K., Campbell, T., & Blazer, G. (1989). Alternative models of the stress buffering hypothesis. *American Journal of Community Psychology, 17*, 625–642.

Larner, A. (1997). The cerebellum in Alzheimer's disease. *Dementia and Geriatric Cognitive Disorder, 8*(4), 203–209.

Lautenschlager, N., Cox, K., Flicker, L., Foster, J., van Bockxmeer, F., Xiao, J., Greenop, K., & Almeida, O. (2008). Effect of physical activity on cognitive function in older adults at risk for Alzheimer disease. *Journal of the American Medical Association, 300*(9),1027–1037.

Lazarus, A. (1989). *The Practice of Multimodal Therapy: Systematic, Comprehensive, and Effective Psychotherapy*. Baltimore, Maryland: Johns Hopkins University Press.

Lee, Y., Tabourne, C.E.S., & Yoon, J. (2008a). Effects of life review program on emotional well-being of Korean elderly with Alzheimer's disease. *American Journal of Recreation Therapy, 7*(3), 35–45.

Lee, Y., Tabourne, C. E. S., & Yoon, J. (2008b). Life review program as a therapeutic recreation intervention for Korean elderly with Alzheimer's disease: Qualitative analysis. *Annual in Therapeutic Recreation, 16,* 171–180.

Lemonick, M.D., & Park, A. (2001, May 14). The Nun Study: How one scientist and 678 sisters are helping unlock the secrets of Alzheimer's. *Time Magazine,* 55–64.

Lepper, M.R., & Woolverton, M. (2002). The wisdom of practice: Lessons learned from the study of highly effective tutors. In J. Aronson (Ed.), *Improving academic achievement: Impact of psychological factors on education* (pp. 135–158). Orlando, FL: Academic Press.

Levine Madori, L. (2007). *Therapeutic thematic arts programming for older adults.* Baltimore, MD: Health Professions Press.

Levine Madori, L. (2009a). *Alzheimer's disease, cognitive functioning and psychosocial well-being.* Germany: VMD Publishing.

Levine Madori, L. (2009b). Uses of therapeutic thematic arts programming, TTAP Method, for enhanced cognitive and psychosocial functioning in the geriatric population. *American Journal of Recreational Therapy, 8*(1).

Levine Madori, L. (2009c). *Cognitive and psychosocial functioning in residents with Alzheimer's disease: Therapeutic recreation participation correlated to improved cognition and quality of life in those residents living in a skilled nursing facility.* Doctoral dissertation. Saarbrücken, Germany: VDM Verlag.

Levine Madori, L., Sherrier, C., Grable, S., Hanley, C., Walsh, L., & Martinez, A. (2010). Use of TTAP Method with residents in Northern Manor dementia unit. Unpublished research methods.

Li, R. (1996). *A theory of conceptual intelligence: Thinking, learning, creativity and giftedness.* Westport, CT: Praeger.

Linnenbrink, E.A., & Pintrich, P.A. (2004). Role of affect in change processing in academic contexts. In D. Y. Dai & R. J. Sternberg (Eds.), *Motivation, emotion, and cognition: Integrative perspectives on intellectual functioning and development* (pp. 57–88). Mahwah, NJ: Lawrence Erlbaum Associates.

LoboPrabhu, S., Molinari, V., & Lomax J. (2007). The transitional object in dementia: Clinical observations. *International Journal of Applied Psychoanalytic Studies, 4*(2), 144–169.

Lycan, W.G., (Ed.). (1999). *Mind and cognition: An anthology* (2nd ed.). Malden, MA: Blackwell.

Malchiodi, C. (2003). *Handbook of art therapy.* New York: Guilford Press.

Manly, J., Tang, M., Schupf, N., & Stern., Y. (2005). Implementing diagnostic criteria and estimating frequency of mild cognitive impairment in an urban community. *Archives of Neurology, 62,* 1739–1746.

Markova, I., & Berrios, G. (2001). The "object" of insight assessment: Relationship to insight "structure." *Psychopathology, 34,* 245–252.

Mastel-Smith, B., Binder, B., Malecha, A., Hersch, G., Symes, L., & McFarlane, J. (2006). Testing therapeutic life review offered by home care workers to decrease depression among home-dwelling older women. *Issues in Mental Health Nursing, 27,* 1037–1049.

McClellan, T. (2001). Study and analysis of cognitive, motivational and group treatment of alcoholics through brain imaging. *Journal of American Medical Association, 9,* 50–56.

McEwen, B.S., & Sapolsky, R.M. (1995). Stress and cognitive function. *Current Opinion in Neurobiology, 5*(2), 205s–216.

McKenzie, E. (1996). The Cultural Life Review Program for African-American seniors. *Activities Director's Quarterly for Alzheimer's & Other Dementia Patients, 7*(3), 1–19. Available at http://www.citra.org/Assets/documents/Sirey%20proposal.pdf

McKenzie, R. (2008). An ailing brain with imagination undimmed. *BBC News.* Available at http://news.bbc.co.uk/2/hi/uk_news/magazine/7560713.stm

McKinney, C.H., Antoni, M.H., Kumar, M., Tims, F.C., & McCabe, P.M. (1997). Effects of guided imagery and music (GIM) therapy on mood and cortisol in healthy adults, *Journal of Health Psychology, 16*(4), 390–400.

McPherson, A., Furniss, F., Sdogati, C., Cesaroni, F., Tartaglini, B., & Lindesay, J. (2001). Effects of individualized memory aids on the conversation of persons with severe dementia: A pilot study. *Aging & Mental Health, 5*(3), 289–294.

Meara, E., Richards, S., & Cutler, D. (2008). The gap gets bigger: Changes in mortality and life expectancy, by education, 1981–2000. *Health Affairs, 27*(2), 350–360.

Meyer, D.K., & Turner, J.C. (2002). Discovering emotion in classroom motivation research. *Educational Psychologist, 37,* 107–114.

Moniz-Cook, E., Agar, S., Gibson, G., Win, T., & Wing, M. (1998). A preliminary study of the effects of early intervention with people with dementia and their families in a memory clinic. *Aging & Mental Health, 2*(3), 199–211.

Moody, E.F. (2009). Life expectancy tables. Available at http://www.efmoody.com/estate/lifeexpectancy.html

Morano, C., & Bravo, M. (2002). A psychoeducational model for Hispanic Alzheimer's disease caregivers. *Gerontologist, 42,* 122–126.

Mori, E., Ikeda, M., Hirono, N., Kitagaki, H., Imamura, T., & Shimomura, T. (1999). Amygdalar volume and emotional memory in Alzheimer's disease. *American Journal of Psychiatry, 156,* 216–222.

Nagy, Z., Hindley, J., Braak, H., Braak, E., Yilmazer-Hanke, M., Schultz, C., Barnetson, L., King, E., Jobst, K., & Smith, A. (1999). The progression of Alzheimer's disease from limbic regions to the neocortex: Clinical, radiological and pathological relationships. *Dementia and Geriatric Cognitive Disorders,10*(2), 115–120.

National Coalition of Creative Arts Therapies Associations. (2009). Statement of purpose. Available at http://www.nccata.org/

National Institute on Aging. (2005). Progress report on Alzheimer's disease. NIH Publication No. 05-5724. Bethesda, MD: Author. Available at http://www.alzheimers.org/pr04-05/index.asp

National Therapeutic Recreation Society. (1982). Philosophical position statement. Alexandria, VA: Author.

National Therapeutic Recreation Society. (2002). Philosophical position statement. Alexandria, VA: Author. Available at http://www.nrpa.org/

Nelson, A.P. (2005). *The Harvard Medical School guide to achieving optimal memory.* Boston: McGraw-Hill.

Newson, R., & Kemps, E. (2005). General lifestyle activities as a predictor of current cognition and cognitive change in older adults: A cross-sectional and longitudinal examination. *Journals of Gerontology Series B: Psychological Sciences and Social Sciences, 60*, 113–120.

Norman, R. (2000). Cultivating imagination in adult education. Available at http://www.edst.educ.ubc.ca/aerc/2000/normanr-final.PDF

Ofstedal, B., Plassman, L., Langa, M., Fisher, G., Herringa, G., Weir, R., et al. (2007). Prevalence of dementia in the United States: The Aging Demographic and Memory Study. *Neuroepidemiology, 29, 125*–132.

Orlando, P. (2006). Mnemosyne: A goddess for storytelling, creativity and reading comprehension. storytelling, memory, and learning. *Educational Horizons, 84*(3). Available at http://www.pilambda.org/horizons/v84-3/balance.pdf

Ornstein, E., & Ganzer, C. (2000). Strengthening the strengths perspective: An integrative relational approach. *Psychoanalytic Social Work, 7*(3), 57–78.

Orrell, M., Butler, R., & Bebbington, P. (2000). Social factors and the outcome of dementia. *International Journal of Geriatric Psychiatry, 15*(6), 515–520.

Ostbye, T., Krause, K., Norton, M., Tschanz, J., & Sanders, L. (2006). Ten dimensions of health and their relationships with overall self-reported health and survival in a predominately religiously active elderly population: The Cache County Memory Study. *Journal of the American Geriatric Society, 54*, 199–209.

Papp, P., & Imber-Black, E. (2004). Family themes: Transmission and transformation. *Family Process, 35*(1), 5–20.

Perese, E., Simon, M., Ryan, E., Kverno, K., Rabins, P., Blass, D., Hicks, L., & Black, B. (2008). Prevalence and treatment of neuropsychiatric symptoms in advanced dementia. *Journal Gerontology Nursing, 34*(12), 8–15.

Perry, B.D. (2001). The neurodevelopmental impact of violence in childhood. In D. Schetky & E. P. Benedek (Eds.), *Textbook of child and adolescent forensic psychiatry* (pp. 221–238). Washington, DC: American Psychiatric Press.

Perry, B.D. (2006). Applying principles of neurodevelopment to clinical work with maltreated and traumatized children: The neurosequential model of therapeutics. In B. Webb (Ed.), *Working with traumatized youth in child welfare.* New York: Guilford Press.

Perry, B.D. (2008, November 19). Healing impact of art therapy on brain functioning of children who have suffered trauma and neglect. Bruce Perry Keynote Address presented at the annual conference of the American Art Therapy Association. Cleveland, OH.

Perry, B.D. (2009). Examining child maltreatment through a neurodevelopmental lens: clinical application of the Neurosequential Model of Therapeutics. *Journal of Loss and Trauma, 14*, 240–255.

Perry, B.D., & Hambrick, E. (2008). The neurosequential model of therapeutics. *Reclaiming Children and Youth, 17*(3), 38–43.

Perry, B.D., Pollard, R.A., Blakely, T.L., Baker, W.L., & Vigilante, D. (1995). Childhood trauma, the neurobiology of adaptation, and "use-dependent" development of the brain. How "states" become "traits." *Infant Mental Health Journal, 16*, 271–291.

Peterson, C.A., & Gunn, S.L. (1984). *Therapeutic recreation program design: Principles and procedures.* Englewood Cliffs, NJ: Prentice Hall.

Phelps, E. (2004). Human emotion and memory: Interactions of the amygdala and hippocampal complex. *Current Opinion in Neurobiology, 14*(2), 198–202.

Pignatti, F., Rozzini, R., & Trabucchi, M. (2002). Physical activity and cognitive decline in elderly persons. *Archives of Internal Medicine, 162,* 361–362.

Pizarro, J. (2004). The efficacy of art and writing therapy: Increasing positive mental health outcomes and participant retention after exposure to traumatic experience. *Journal of the American Art Therapy Association, 21*(1), 5–12.

Pruessner, J.C., Lord, C., Meaney, M., & Lupien, S. (2004). Effects of self-esteem on age-related changes in cognition and the regulation of the hypothalamic-pituitary-adrenal axis. *Annals of the New York Academy of Sciences, 1032,* 186–190.

Reifler, B., & Larson, E. (1990). Excess disability in dementia of the Alzheimer's type. In E. Light & B. Leibowitz (Eds.), *Alzheimer's disease treatment and family stress.* New York, NY: Hemesphire.

Reisberg, D., & Heuer, F. (1992). Remembering the details of emotional events. In E. Winograd & U. Neisser (Eds.), *Affect and accuracy in recall: Studies of "flashbulb" memories* (pp. 162–190). Cambridge: Cambridge University Press.

Reisberg, B., & Kluger, A. (1998). Assessing the progression of dementia: Diagnostic considerations. In C. Salzman (Ed.), *Clinical geriatric psychopharmacology* (pp. 432–462). Baltimore, MD: Williams & Wilkins.

Reisberg, B., Ferris, S. H., de Leon, M. J., & Crook, T. (1982). The Global Deterioration Scale for assessment of primary degenerative dementia. *American Journal of Psychiatry, 139,* 1136–1139.

Reisberg, B., Ferris, S. H., Leon, M.J., & Crook, T. (1982). The Global Deterioration Scale for assessment of primary degenerative dementia. *American Journal of Psychiatry, 139,* 1136–1139.

Reisberg, B., Ferris, S.H., Finkel, S., & Overall, J.E. (1998). The Activities of Daily Living International Scale (ADL-IS): History and progress. Abstract. *European Archives of Psychiatry and Clinical Neuroscience, 248,* (Suppl. 1), S4–S5.

Rentz, C. (2002). Memories in the Making©: Outcome-based evaluation of an art based program for individuals with dementing illnesses. *American Journal of Alzheimer's Disease and Other Dementias, 17*(3), 175–181.

Richards, M. (2004). The cognitive consequences of concealing feelings. *Current Directions in Psychological Science, 13*(4), 131–134.

Rogers, C. (1961). *On becoming a person: A therapist's view of psychotherapy.* Boston: Houghton Mifflin.

Rosenberg, M. (1965). *Society and the adolescent self-image.* Princeton, NJ: Princeton University Press.

Rovio, S., Kåreholt, I., Helkala, E., Viitanen, M., Winblad, B., Tuomilehto, J., Soininen, H., Nissinen, A., & Kivipelto, M. (2005). Leisure-time physical activity at midlife and the risk of dementia and Alzheimer's disease. *Lancet Neurology, 4*(11), 705–711.

Rowan, J. (2001). *Ordinary ecstasy: The dialectics of humanistic psychology.* London: Brunner Routledge.

Ryan, E. (2006). Finding a new voice. *Journal of Language and Social Psychology, 25*(4), 423–436.

Sabat, S. (2006). Implicit memory and people with Alzheimer's disease: Implication for caregiving. *American Journal of Alzheimer's Disease and Other Dementias, 21*(1), 11–14.

Scarmeas, N., Stern, Y. (2003). Cognitive reserve and lifestyle. *Journal of Clinical & Experimental Neuropsychology, 25,* 625–633.

Scarmeas, N., Levy, G., Tang, M.-X., Manly, J., & Stern, Y. (2001). Influence of leisure activity on the incidence of Alzheimer's disease. *Neurology, 57,* 2236–2242.

Schindler, R., & Cucio, C. (2000). Late-life dementia. Review of the APA guidelines for patient management. *Geriatrics, 55*(10), 55–60.

Schuit, A.J., Feskens, E.J., Launer, L.J., & Kromhout, D. (2001). Physical activity and cognitive decline: The role of apoliproprotein e4 allele. *Medicine and Science in Sports and Exercise, 33,* 772–777.

Schwarzer, R., & Jerusalem, M. (1995). Generalized Self-Efficacy Scale. In S. Weinman & M. Johnson (Eds.), *Measures in health psychology: A user's portfolio. Causal and control beliefs* (pp. 35–37). Windsor, UK: Nefer-Nelson.

Serrano, C., Allegri, R., Martelli, M., Taragano, F., & Rinalli, P. (2005). Visual art, creativity and dementia. *Vertex, 16*(64), 418–429. Available at http://www.ncbi.nlm.nih.gov/pubmed/16314895

Shapiro, D., Hardy, G., Aldridge, J., Davidson, C., Rowe, C., & Reilly, S. (1999). Therapist responsiveness to client attachment styles and issues observed in client-identified significant events in psychodynamic-interpersonal psychotherapy. *Psychotherapy Research, 9*(1), 36–53.

Sheikh, J.I., & Yesavage, J.A. (1986). Geriatric Depression Scale (GDS): Recent evidence and development of a shorter version. *Clinical Gerontology, 5,* 165–173.

Shulman, K., Shedletsky, R., & Silver, I. (1986). The challenge of time: Clock drawing and cognitive function in the elderly. *International Journal of Geriatric Psychiatry, 1,* 135–140.

Sloane, P.D., Hoeffer, B., Mitchell, C.M., McKenzie, D.A., Barrick, A.L., Rader, J., Stewart, B.J., Talerico, K.A., Rasin, J.H., Zink, R.C., & Koch, G.G. (2004). Effect of person-centered showering and the towel bath on bathing-associated aggression, agitation, and discomfort in nursing home residents with dementia: A randomized, controlled trial. *Journal of the American Geriatrics Society, 52*(11), 1795–1804.

Snowdon, D. (2001). *Aging with grace: What the Nun Study teaches us about leading longer, healthier, and more meaningful lives.* New York: Bantam Books.

Snowdon, D., Kemper, S., Mortimer, J., Greiner, L., Wekstein D., & Markesbery, W. (1996). Linguistic ability in early life and cognitive function and Alzheimer's disease in late life: Findings from the Nun Study. *Journal of the American Medical Association, 275,* 528–532.

Sperner-Unterweger, B. (2000*). Psychoneuroimmunology: Hypotheses and current research, 6th expert meeting on psychoimmunology.* Basel, Switzerland: S. Karger AG.

Steffens, D.C., Otey E., Alexopoulos, G.S., Butters, M., Cuthbert, B., Ganguli, M., et al. (2006). Perpectives on depression, mild cognitive impairment and cognitive decline. *Archives of General Psychiatry, 63,* 130–138.

Stein, D., & Hoffman, S. (2003). Concepts of CNS plasticity in the context of brain damage and repair. *Journal of Head Trauma Rehabilitation, 18,* 317–341.

Sterin, J. (2002). Essay on a word: A lived experience of Alzheimer's disease. *Dementia, 1*(1), 7–10.

Stern, Y., Albert, S., Tang, M-X., & Tsai, W-Y. (1999). Rate of memory decline in AD is related to education and occupation: Cognitive reserve? *Neurology, 53,* 1942–1947.

Stern, Y., Gurland, B., Tatemichi, T., Tang, M.X., Wilder, D., & Mayeux, R. (1994). Influence of education and occupation on the incidence of Alzheimer's disease. *Journal of the American Medical Association, 271,* 1004–1010.

Stern, Y., Moeller, J.R., & Anderson, K.E. (2000). Different brain networks mediate task performance in normal aging and Alzheimer's disease: Defining compensation. *Neurology, 55,* 1291–1297.

Sunderland, T., Hill, L., Mellow, M., Lawlor, B.A., Gundersheimer, J., Newhouse, P.A., & Grafman, J.H. (1989). Clock drawing in Alzheimer's disease: A novel measure of dementia severity. *Journal of the American Geriatric Society, 37*(8), 725–729.

Tabourne, C.E.S. (1991). The effects of a life review recreation therapy program on confused nursing home residents. *Topics in Geriatric Rehabilitation, 7*(2), 13–21.

Tabourne, C.E.S. (1995a). The benefits of a life review program for a patient newly admitted to a nursing home: A case study. *Therapeutic Recreation Journal, 29*(3), 228–236.

Tabourne, C. (1995b). The effects of a life review program on disorientation, social interaction, and self-esteem of nursing home residents. *International Journal of Aging and Human Development, 41*(3), 251–266.

Tang, M., Cross, P., Andrews, H., Jacobs, M., Small, S., Bell, K., et al. (2001). Incidence of AD in African-Americans, Caribbean Hispanics, and Caucasians in northern Manhattan. *American Academy of Neurology, 56,* 49–56.

Tarbuck, A.F., & Paykel, E.S. (1995). Effects of major depression on the cognitive function of younger and older subjects. *Psychological Medicine, 25*(2), 285–296.

Terri, L., Gibbons, E., McCurry, M., Logsdog, G., Bucher, M., Barlow, E., Kukull, A., et al. (2003). Exercise plus behavioral management in patients with Alzheimer's disease. *Journal of the American Medical Association, 290*(15), 2015–2022.

Thompson, P. (2003). Surface-based analysis of the study and function of the human cerebral cortex. Brain mapping research program at the University of California, Los Angeles. Available at http://Faculty.Washington.edu/chudler/image.html.

Tornstam, L. (1999). Gerotranscendence and the functions of reminiscence. *Journal of Aging and Identity, 4*(3), 155–166.

Tornstam, L. (2005). *Gerotranscendence: A developmental theory of positive aging.* New York: Springer.

Trevarthen, C. (1990). *Brain circuits and functions of the mind.* New York: Cambridge University Press.

Truscott, M. (2004). Adapting leisure and creative activities for people with early stage dementias. *Alzheimer's Care Quarterly, 5*(2), 92–102.

University of California–Irvine. (2007, January 24). Learning slows physical progression of Alzheimer's disease. *ScienceDaily.* Available at http://www.sciencedaily.com/releases/2007/01/070123182024.htm

University of California–San Diego. (2009, December 28). Alzheimer's: How amyloid beta reduces plasticity related to synaptic signaling. *ScienceDaily.* Available at http://www.sciencedaily.com/releases/2009/12/091228152352.htm

U.S. Census Bureau. (2011). The older population: 2010. Washington, DC: U.S. Department of Commerce, Economics and Statistics Administration.

Voelkl, J.E., Galecki, A.T., & Fries, B.E. (1996). Nursing home residents with severe cognitive impairments: Predictors of participation in activity groups. *Therapeutic Recreation Journal, 30*(1), 27–40.

Voelkl, J.E., & Mathieu, M. (1995). Intra-individual variation in the subjective experiences of older adults in a nursing home. *Therapeutic Recreation Journal, 29*(2), 114–123.

Wadensten, B., & Carlsson, M. (2001). A qualitative study of nursing staff members' interpretations of signs of gerotranscendence. *Journal of Advanced Nursing, 36*(5), 635–642.

Washington University. (August 1998). One intelligence or many? Alternative approaches to cognitive abilities. Available at http://www.personalityresearch.org/papers/paik.html

Wechsler, D. (1981). Wechsler Adult Intelligence Scale—Revised. New York: Psychological Corp.

Willis, S., Tennstedt, S., Marsiske, M., Ball, K., Elias, J., Koepke, K., Morris, J., Rebok, G., Unverzagt, F., Stoddard, A., & Wright, E. (2006). Longterm effects of cognitive training on everyday functional outcomes in older adults. *Journal of the American Medical Association, 296*(23), 2852–2854.

Wilson, L.O. (2006). Beyond Bloom—A new version of the cognitive taxonomy. Available at http://www4.uwsp.edu/education/lwilson/curric/newtaxonomy.htm

Wong, P.T., and Watt, L.M. (1991). What types of reminiscence are associated with successful aging? *Psychology and Aging, 6,* 272–279.

Woods, B., Spector, A., Jones, C., Orrell, M., & Davis, S. (2005). Reminiscence therapy for dementia: A review. *Cochrane Database of Systematic Reviews,* Issue 2.

Yaakov, S. (2007). *Cognitive reserve: Theory and application.* New York: Taylor & Frances.

Yankner, B. (2000, March). A century of cognitive decline. *Nature, 404,* 125.

Yu, F., Rose, K., Burgener, S., Cunningham, C., Buettner, L., Beattie, E., Bossen, A., Buckwalter, K., Fick, D., Fitzsimmons, S., Kolanowski, A., Janet, K., Specht, P., Richeson, N., Testad, I., & McKenzie, S. (2009). Cognitive training for early-stage Alzheimer's disease and dementia. *Journal of Gerontology Nursing, 35*(3), 23–29.

Zanetti, O., Binetti, G., Magni, E., Rozzini, L., Bianchetti, A., & Trabucchi, M. (1997). Procedural memory stimulation in Alzheimer's disease: Impact of a training programme. *Acta Neurologica Scandinavica, 95,* 152–157.

Zarit, H., Femia, D., Watson, J., Rice-Oeschger, L., & Kakas, B. (2004). Memory club: A group intervention for people with early-stage dementia and their care partners. *Gerontologist, 44*(2), 262–269.

Zatz, M.M., & Goldstein, A.L. (1985). Thymosins, lumphokines and the immunology of aging, *Gerontology, 31*(4), 263–277.

Index

Note: *b* indicates boxes, *f* indicates figures, *t* indicates tables.

Acetylcholine, 94
Activities and activity level
   flow and, 31
   importance of, 123–124, 125–126, 134
   learning systems and, 108, 109
   mild cognitive impairment (MCI)
     and, 15–16
Activities of daily living, 12, 14, 15, 22–23
Affective system of learning, 107, 107*b*,
  108
Aggression, 80
Aging, normal, 11–13, 21
Aging theories
   Continuum of Psychological
     Domains, 127–131, 128*t*
   gerotranscendence, 146–149
   life-span approach, 124–126, 127
   stages/tasks of life, 122–124
Alzheimer's disease
   brain and, 7, 8*f*, 9, 10*f*, 11, 14, 92*f*,
     93–94, 96–97, 98–99
   care/intervention, *see* Alzheimer's
     disease care/intervention
   delaying, *see* Alzheimer's disease
     delay/prevention
   dementia diagnosis and, 94
   depression and, 99
   losses with diagnosis of, 101
   needs/capabilities with, 29–31, 30*f*,
     109–110, 110*f*, 136
   nonnormative influences and,
     124–125
   prevalence of, 7, 43
   progression of, 14–17, 17*f*
   stages of, *see* Alzheimer's disease
     stages
   stress and, 100
   warning signs of, 11–13

Alzheimer's disease care/intervention
   Continuum of Psychological Domains
     and, 129–131
   delaying, *see* Alzheimer's disease
     delay/prevention
   ego integrity and, 127
   families and TTAP Method, 15–17,
     16*f*, 17*f*, 18*f*, 19
   life review and, 131–135, 134*f*
   needs of older adults and, 109–110,
     110*f*, 136
   object relations theory and, 141
   person-centered therapy, 121,
     135–138, 161–162
   self-growth and, 122–123
   stimulation of memory and, 19
   TTAP Method, *see* TTAP Method
     with Alzheimer's disease; *specific*
     Alzheimer's stages
Alzheimer's disease delay/prevention
   brain stimulation, 90
   cardiovascular activity, 66
   communication, 18*f*
   early intervention, 100–101
   family participation, 16
   memory stimulation and, 113
   multimodal approaches and, 39
   psychosocial interventions, 46, 96–99
   review/reminiscence and, 84
   risk factors, 89
   TTAP Method, 101–102
   see also TTAP Method with
     Alzheimer's disease
Alzheimer's disease stages
   beta amyloid plaques/tangles and, 9,
     96–97, 98–99
   brain regions and, 10*f*, 92*f*, 93–94
   memory and, 21–24, 53

Alzheimer's disease stages *(continued)*
    overview of, 9, 10*f*, 13, 21–24
    progression to, 14–15
    survival rates and, 100–101
    see also specific stages
Analysis ability
    learning and, 104
    in Levine Madori Taxonomy, 150*f*,
       151, 151*f*, 152, 153*f*
Anxiety, 99, 166, 166*f*, 167*f*
Application of learned information
    Bloom's Taxonomy, 104
    Levine Madori Taxonomy, 150*f*, 151,
       151*f*, 152, 153*f*
Art and recreation therapists, 43–44
Arts programming
    balance of ability/challenge in, 35,
       112
    benefits of, 41, 139, 158
Artwork, 61, 62
Assessment, 11, 128–129
    see also Client feedback/evaluation

Balance of ability and challenge, 35, 112
Balls/balloons in movement program, 66
Behavioral symptoms of Alzheimer's
    disease, 9, 11, 23
Bergen Regional Medical Center
    phototherapy project at, 78
    TTAP Method at, 115, 116*t*–117*t*,
       119, 158
Beta amyloid plaques
    Alzheimer's disease and, 9, 96–97,
       98–99
    brain regions and, 93
    learning and, 95
Beta amyloid proteins, 9, 94, 98–99
Biopsychosocial models, 128–129
Bloom's Taxonomy, 103–105, 150, 150*f*,
    151*f*, 153*f*
Brain
    Alzheimer's disease and, 7, 8*f*, 9, 10*f*,
       11, 14, 92*f*, 93–94, 96–97, 98–99
    depression/emotions and cognition, 99
    intelligence and, 107–108
    learning systems of, 106–107, 107*b*
    memory and, 19, 47, 89, 94–95, 110*f*
    regions/functions of, 90–91, 91*f*, 92*f*,
       93–94
    stimulation of, *see* Brain stimulation
    stress and cognition, 100
    see also specific brain regions
Brain stem, 91*f*, 93

Brain stimulation
    Alzheimer's research and, 96–99
    cell regeneration and, 87–90,
       112–113, 130–131
    client feedback on, 115, 119
    cognition and thematic programming,
       107–110, 108*t*, 110*f*
    creativity and, 111–112
    documentation of results, 168, 168*f*,
       169*f*, 170
    early intervention and, 100–101
    emotions and, 110–111, 113
    illustration of regions, 118*f*
    neurosequential model of
       therapeutics (NMT) and, 138–139
    therapeutic implications, 101–102
    TTAP Method steps and, *see* Brain
       stimulation and TTAP Method steps
Brain stimulation and TTAP Method steps
    conversation/communication, 46, 47,
       108*t*, 116*t*–117*t*
    documentation of results, 168, 168*f*,
       169*f*, 170
    drawing/painting, 60, 108*t*, 116*t*–117*t*
    food experiences, 73, 108*t*, 117*t*
    illustration of regions, 118*f*
    learning styles and, 107–108, 108*t*,
       115, 116*t*–117*t*
    movement/dance, 36, 68, 108*t*, 117*t*
    music/meditation, 36, 57, 108*t*,
       116*t*–117*t*
    neurosequential model of
       therapeutics (NMT) and, 138–139,
       140, 140*f*
    phototherapy, 78, 108*t*
    sculpture, 108*t*, 117*t*, 169*f*
    sensory stimulation, 108*t*, 118*f*
    theme events, 76, 107–110, 108*t*,
       110*f*, 118*f*
    writing as group, 71, 108*t*, 117*t*, 169*f*
Brainstorming, 27, 48–49, 50*f*, 51
Broca's area
    description of, 91*f*, 93
    function of, 98
    sculpture and, 169*f*
    see also Brain stimulation and TTAP
       Method steps

Caregiver burden, 9, 11
Categories of objects, 142*f*
Causation patterns, process and, 49, 50*f*
CCDERS Approach
    communication and, 47–48

Continuum of Psychological Domains
and, 128–129
feedback on, 81
Cell regeneration, 87–90, 112–113,
130–131
see also Brain stimulation
Cerebellum
Alzheimer's disease and, 98–99
description of, 91*f*, 93
writing and, 169*f*
Cerebral cortex, 10*f*, 90, 92*f*
Cerebrum, 90, 91*f*
Children in intergenerational programs,
82–84
Choice and freedom, 33
Client feedback/evaluation
on benefits of TTAP Method, 115,
119, 158, 163
flow and, 35
on intergenerational programming, 84
learning style/brain regions and, 108*t*
overview of, 56, 80–82
see also TTAP Method steps
Client verbal feedback
ownership of processes and, 170
quality of life and, 115, 119
well-being and, 80–81
Cognitive functioning
Alzheimer's disease and, 21–24
art activities and, 139, 158
cardiovascular activity and, 66
Continuum of Psychological Domains
and, 130
creativity and, 111
emotions and, 99
life review and, 131–132
neurons and, 88
psychosocial interventions and, 96,
97
reserve and neuroplasticity, 95
stimulation of, 25–26, 113, 119
stress and, 100
themes/brain stimulation and, 107–
110, 108*t*, 110*f*
transcendence and, 154*f*
see also Memory; Mild cognitive
impairment (MCI)
Cognitive reserve, 95
Cognitive stimulation, 25–26, 113, 119
Communication
Alzheimer's disease and, 21–24,
44–45, 47
benefits of, 29, 30*f*

cognitive stimulation and, 119
with family members, 16*f*, 17, 17*f*,
18*f*, 19
as first TTAP Method step, 46–48
flow and, 36
language and, 12, 14, 89, 97
long-term memory and, 18*f*, 19
music therapy and, 37
objects and, 31
processing artwork and, 61, 62
stimulation of, 97
themes and, 138
withdrawal and, 17*f*
Communication breakdown, 44–45, 47
Communication disorder, 44
Competence, sense of, 34
Comprehension level, 104
Concentration/focus, 35
Concept patterns, 49, 50*f*, 51
Confusion of place and time, 12, 14
Context/environment, 144, 144*f*, 165–166
Continuum of Psychological Domains,
127–131, 128*t*, 153, 154*f*
Continuum of wellness, 126
Control, sense of, 34, 35
Conversation
benefits of, 71, 102
brain stimulation and, 46, 47, 108*t*,
116*t*–117*t*
as fundamental TTAP element,
137–138
intergenerational programming in, 82
language and, 12, 14, 89, 97
object relations theory and, 142*f*
overview of, 54, 56–57
person-centered care and, 161
remembering and, 152
see also TTAP Method steps
Counting, 53, 72–73
Creation function, 150*f*, 151, 151*f*, 152,
153*f*
Creative writing, 37–38
see also Writing as group
Creativity
brain stimulation and, 111–112
Food for Thought activity, 54
in Levine Madori Taxonomy, 150*f*,
151, 151*f*, 152, 153*f*
Curiosity, 37–38
Cutting and pasting, 60

Daily living skills, 12, 14, 15, 22–23
Dance, *see* Movement and dance

Declarative/procedural knowledge, 53–54, 73, 109, 110*f*

Delay of Alzheimer's disease, *see* Alzheimer's disease delay/prevention

Dementia
Continuum of Psychological Domains and, 129–131
ego integrity and, 127
health care costs and, 11
memory loss and, 94
person-centered care and, 136
self-growth and, 122–123
see also Alzheimer's disease

Dendrites, 7, 8*f*

Depression, 99, 133, 142*b*

Descriptive patterns, 48–49, 50*f*, 51

Despair, *see* Ego integrity versus despair

Developmental theories, 122–126, 127
see also Aging theories

Development through learning, 37–38

Differentiation of likes/dislikes, 29–30, 30*f*

Disability, excess, 101

Disorientation, *see* Confusion of place and time

Documentation of research on TTAP Method
existing evidence, 157–158
funding opportunities and, 158–159
monetary impact on facility, 170
overview of, 170–171
person-centered care, 161–162
quality of life, 162–163, 164*f*, 165–166, 165*f*, 166*f*, 167*f*, 168, 169*f*, 170
session attendance/duration, 160–161, 160*f*

Drama or theater
intergenerational programming in, 84
learning style/brain regions and, 108*t*
overview of, 56, 80
see also TTAP Method steps

Drawing and painting
brain stimulation and, 60, 108*t*, 116*t*–117*t*
intergenerational programming in, 82
overview of, 55, 59–62, 59*f*, 62*f*
see also TTAP Method steps

Duration and session attendance, 160–161, 160*f*

Early-stage Alzheimer's disease, *see* Mild/early stage Alzheimer's disease

Efficacy beliefs, 33–34

Ego integrity versus despair, 122–123, 127, 131–135, 134*f*

Emotions
artwork and, 60–61, 62
benefits of TTAP Method and, 30, 30*f*, 119
brain stimulation and, 110–111, 113
cognition and, 99
Continuum of Psychological Domains and, 130
importance of expressing, 30, 30*f*, 37–38
life review and, 133
transcendence and, 154*f*
voice in programming and, 80–81

Entorhinal cortex
Alzheimer's disease and, 10*f*, 92*f*, 93, 97, 98
description of, 91*f*, 93

Environment/context, 144, 144*f*, 165–166

Ericksonian stages/tasks of life, 122–124, 127, 131–135, 134*f*

Evaluation ability
learning and, 105
in Levine Madori Taxonomy, 150*f*, 151, 151*f*, 152, 153*f*

Evaluation of TTAP Method, *see* Client feedback/evaluation; Documentation of research on TTAP Method

Excess disability, 101

Facts as theme example, 54

Family members
creative activities and, 111, 112
person-centered care and, 137
theme events and, 74
TTAP Method and, 15–17, 16*f*, 17*f*, 18*f*, 19

Feedback of clients, *see* Client feedback/evaluation

Feelings, *see* Emotions

Financial issues/funding, 11, 158–159, 160

Flow
brain wellness and, 111–112
descriptive patterning and, 51
gerotranscendence and, 149
guided imagery example, 142*b*
skill/challenge match and, 31
TTAP Method and, 26, 34–36

Food experiences
brain stimulation and, 73, 108*t*, 117*t*
intergenerational programming in, 83

memory stimulation and, 53–54
   overview of, 55, 71–73, 72*f*
   see also TTAP Method steps
Food for Thought activity, 54
Foundations of TTAP Method, *see* Brain
   stimulation; Learning and intelligence;
   Theories underlying TTAP Method
Freedom and choice, 33
Frontal lobes, 90–91, 91*f*, 98, 169*f*
Frustration of family members, 17, 17*f*
Funding/financial issues, 11, 158–159, 160

Garden theme
   for drawing/painting, 60
   for food experiences, 71
   guided imagery example with, 57, 58,
      142*b*
   movement/dance and, 68
   sculpture example with, 63
   for sensory stimulation, 79
   theme event on, 75
Gardner, Howard, 105–107, 106*t*, 108*t*
Generalization patterns, 49, 50*f*
Gerotranscendence, 146–149
Goal/feedback clarity, 35
Graphic organizing tools, 48–49, 50*f*, 51–53
Group experiences
   artwork processing, 61–62
   benefits of, 29, 30, 30*f*
   culture and, 44–45
   theme-centered interaction theory
      (TCI) and, 143–146, 144*f*
Guided imagery and music
   exercise examples, 57, 58*b*, 142*b*
   intergenerational programming in, 82
   learning style/brain regions and,
      116*t*–117*t*
   theme-centered interaction theory
      (TCI) and, 146

Health care costs, 11
Helplessness, learned, 45
Hippocampus
   Alzheimer's disease and, 10*f*, 92*f*,
      93–94, 97, 98
   cell regeneration and, 112, 113
   description of, 91*f*, 93
   emotions and, 110–111
Humanistic psychology, 135–138

Identity, 132–133, 147
Imagery, *see* Guided imagery and music;
   Visual images

Incontinence, 23, 24
Individualization in TTAP Method, 27,
   145–146
Individual learners, 106*t*
Intelligence, *see* Learning and intelligence
Intense involvement, 35
Interaction, 153, 153*f*
   see also Social relationships
Interests of older adults, 121, 147
   see also Intrinsic motivation
Intergenerational programming, 82–84
Interpersonal learners, 106*t*
Intrapersonal learners, 106*t*
Intrinsic motivation
   flow and, 35
   self-esteem and, 28, 33, 115, 119
   TTAP Method and, 121

Joy, self-expression of, 30, 30*f*
Judgment, decreased or poor, 12, 15

Kinesthetic learners, 106*t*
Knowledge
   learning level, 104
   procedural, 53–54, 73, 109, 110*f*

Language
   Alzheimer's disease and, 12, 14
   as predictor of late functioning, 89
   stimulation of, 97
   see also Communication; Conversation
Late-stage Alzheimer's disease, *see* Severe/
   late-stage Alzheimer's disease
Learned helplessness, 45
Learning and intelligence
   beta amyloid plaques and, 95
   Bloom's levels of, 103–105
   continual cognitive stimulation and,
      113
   development through, 37–38
   Gardner's styles/systems of, 105–107,
      106*t*, 107*b*, 108*t*
   Levine Madori Taxonomy on, 150,
      150*f*, 151, 151*f*, 152, 153*f*
   TTAP Method steps/brain region and,
      107–108, 108*t*, 109, 115, 116*t*–117*t*
Leisure activities, *see* Activities and activity
   level
Levine Madori Taxonomy, 149–155, 150*f*,
   151*f*, 153*f*, 154*f*
Life review
   Alzheimer's disease and, 84, 131–135,
      134*f*

Life review   *(continued)*
    benefits of, 38, 84, 147
    ego integrity and, 123
    well-being and, 25
    see also Reminiscence
Life Review Program (LRP), 132
Life-span theories, 124–126, 127
Life stories, 37–38, 70
Linguistic learners, 106*t*
Logical learners, 106*t*
Long-term memory
    benefits of recall, 30, 30*f,* 31, 108–109,
        113
    communication and, 18*f,* 19
    music and, 36
    see also Memory
Losing/misplacing things, 12
Loss or sorrow, 62
LRP, *see* Life Review Program
Lucidity, windows of, 45–46

MCI, *see* Mild cognitive impairment
Meditation
    benefits of, 163, 165–166, 165*f*
    needs of older adults for, 148
    overview of, 55, 57, 58*b*
    see also Music and meditation
Memory
    age-related changes in, 11–13
    Alzheimer's disease stages and,
        21–24, 53
    benefits of recall, 30, 30*f,* 31, 108–109,
        110*f,* 113
    brain and, 19, 47, 89, 94–95, 110*f*
    cardiovascular activity and, 66
    communication and, 18*f,* 19
    emotions and, 110–111
    music and, 36
    procedural, 53–54, 73, 109, 110*f*
    stimulation of, 19, 53–54, 113
    story telling and, 37–38
    stress and, 100
    TTAP Method benefits to, 166, 167*f,*
        168
Memory stimulation, 19, 53–54, 113
Mental status examinations, 11
Mice brain research, 87–88, 95
Mid-stage Alzheimer's disease, *see*
    Moderate/mid-stage Alzheimer's
    disease
Mild cognitive decline stage, 21
Mild cognitive impairment (MCI), 15–16,
    96, 142*b*

Mild/early stage Alzheimer's disease
    description of, 9, 10*f,* 14
    life review and, 131
    prevention of progression and, 16
    theme-centered interaction theory
        (TCI) and, 145–146
    therapeutic recreation and, 127
    TTAP Method steps and, *see* Mild/
        early stage Alzheimer's disease and
        TTAP Method steps
Mild/early stage Alzheimer's disease and
    TTAP Method steps
    client feedback, 81–82
    communication, 47
    conversation, 56–57
    drama/theater, 80
    drawing/painting, 59–60
    food experience, 71–72
    movement/dance, 66–68
    music and meditation, 57, 58*b*
    phototherapy, 76–78
    sculpture, 63
    sensory stimulation, 79
    theme events, 75
    writing in groups, 69–70
Mirror use, 166, 168
Moderately severe cognitive decline stage,
    22
Moderate/mid-stage Alzheimer's disease
    description of, 9, 10*f,* 14, 16*f,* 22
    life review and, 133
    memory and, 53
    therapeutic recreation and, 127
    TTAP Method benefits with, 115, 119
    TTAP Method steps and, *see*
        Moderate/mid-stage Alzheimer's
        disease and TTAP Method steps
Moderate/mid-stage Alzheimer's disease
    and TTAP Method steps
    at Bergen Regional Medical Center,
        115, 116*t*–117*t,* 119, 158
    client feedback, 81–82
    drama/theater, 80
    drawing/painting, 59–60
    food experiences, 72
    movement/dance, 68
    phototherapy, 78
    sculpture, 63–64
    sensory stimulation, 79
    theme events, 75
    writing in groups, 70–71
Mood, 13, 133, 164*f,* 165
Motivation, *see* Intrinsic motivation

Motor cortex, 91, 91*f*, 169*f*
Movement and dance
    brain stimulation and, 36, 68, 108*t*,
        117*t*
    overview of, 55, 65–68, 65*f*
    see also TTAP Method steps
Movers/kinesthetic learners, 106*t*
Multicultural groups, 44–45
Multiple intelligences/styles of learning,
    105–107, 106*t*, 108*t*
Musical instruments, 67
Musical learners, 106*t*
Music and meditation
    benefits of, 163, 165–166, 165*f*
    brain stimulation and, 36, 57, 108*t*,
        116*t*–117*t*
    communication and, 37
    guided imagery examples, 57, 58*b*,
        142*b*
    intergenerational programming in, 82
    needs of older adults and, 148
    overview of, 55, 57, 58*b*
    person-centered care and, 161
    theme-centered interaction theory
        (TCI) and, 146
    see also TTAP Method steps

NDT, *see* Neuro-developmental treatment
Needs of older adults
    with Alzheimer's disease, 29–31, 30*f*,
        109–110, 110*f*, 136
    benefits of TTAP Method and, 119
    for solitary meditation, 148
    see also Theories underlying TTAP
        Method
Neocortex, 90–91, 91*f*, 94–95, 97
Neuro-developmental treatment (NDT),
    138
Neurofibrillary tangles, 96–97, 98–99
Neurons
    Alzheimer's disease and, 7, 8*f*
    cell regeneration and, 87–90,
        112–113, 130–131
    cognitive activity and, 88
    see also Brain
Neuroplasticity
    cognitive reserve and, 95
    dendrites and, 7
    TTAP Method benefits to, 138–139,
        140, 140*f*
Neurosequential model of therapeutics
    (NMT) approach, 138–139, 140, 140*f*
Neurotransmitters, 94

NMT, *see* Neurosequential model of
    therapeutics (NMT) approach
Nonnormative/normative influences,
    124–125
Nonverbal communication, 37
Normal aging, 11–13, 21
Normative/nonnormative influences,
    124–125
Northern Manor study
    attendance results, 159–161, 160*f*
    overview of, 158
    quality of life results, 162–163, 164*f*,
        165–166, 165*f*, 166*f*, 167*f*, 168,
        169*f*, 170
Nun Study, 89, 125

Object(s)
    communication and, 31
    drama/theater and, 66, 80
    Food for Thought activity, 54
    life review and, 133–134, 134*f*
    in movement programs, 66
    object relations theory on, 141, 142*b*,
        142*f*, 143
    windows of lucidity and, 45
Object relations theory, 141, 142*b*, 142*f*,
    143
Occipital lobe, 91, 91*f*
    see also Brain stimulation and TTAP
        Method steps
Organizing tools, graphic, 48–49, 50*f*,
    51–53
Orientation, 12, 14, 18*f*

Painting, *see* Drawing and painting
Parietal lobe, 91, 91*f*
Parkinson's disease, 36–37
Past events and communication, 18*f*
Patterning, descriptive, 48–49, 50*f*, 51
People in relation to communication,
    16*f*, 17
Perceived freedom, 33
Personal choice, 33
Personal control, 34, 35
Personality, 13, 23
Person-centered care, 121, 135–138,
    161–162
Person in relation to communication,
    16*f*, 17
Phototherapy
    brain stimulation and, 78, 108*t*
    intergenerational programming in, 83
    life review/reminiscence and, 38

Phototherapy *(continued)*
    overview of, 55, 76–78, 77*f*
    see also TTAP Method steps
Physical functioning
    Continuum of Psychological Domains
        and, 130
    ego integrity and, 123
    stamina results, 167*f,* 168
    transcendence and, 154*f*
Places
    communication about, 16*f,* 17
    confusion of, 12, 14
    flow and, 35
Planning by older adults, 11–12
Plaques, *see* Beta amyloid plaques
Plasticity, 7
    see also Neuroplasticity
Poetry, 37–38
    see also Writing as group
Present events and communication, 18*f*
Prevention of Alzheimer's disease, *see*
    Alzheimer's disease delay/prevention
Problem solving, 11–12, 49, 50*f*
Procedural memory, 53–54, 73, 109,
    110*f*
Process and causation patterns, 49, 50*f*
Props, 66, 80
    see also Object(s)
Proteins, beta amyloid, 9, 94, 98–99
Psychological development, *see*
    Developmental theories
Psychological Domains, Continuum of,
    127–131, 128*t,* 153, 154*f*
Psychology, humanistic, 135–138
Psychosocial interventions, 46, 96–99

Quality of life
    client feedback on, 115, 119
    documentation of, 162–163, 164*f,*
        165–166, 165*f,* 166*f,* 167*f,* 168,
        169*f,* 170
    social relationships and, 39

Recall benefits
    brain stimulation, 108, 109, 110*f,* 113
    in CCDERS Approach, 30, 30*f,* 31
    see also Life review; Memory
Recognition system, 107, 107*b,* 109
Recreation, 126–127
    see also Activities and activity level
Regeneration of brain cells, 87–90,
    112–113, 130–131
    see also Brain stimulation

Reimbursement, Medicare/Medicaid
    policies and documentation, 158–160
Relaxation, 165–166, 165*f*
Remembering, 150, 150*f,* 151*f,* 153*f*
    see also Memory
Reminiscence
    benefits of, 38, 84, 113, 147
    depression and, 133
    helplessness and, 45
    see also Life review
Research on TTAP Method, *see*
    Documentation of research on TTAP
    Method
Resentment of family members, 17, 17*f*
Reticular formation, 91*f,* 93
    see also Brain stimulation and TTAP
        Method steps
Role-playing, 80

Scarves in movement programs, 66–67
Sculpture
    brain stimulation and, 108*t,* 117*t,* 169*f*
    overview of, 55, 63–65, 63*f,* 64*f*
    see also TTAP Method steps
Seashell theme, 45–46
Seasons as theme example
    sensory stimulation, 79
    TTAP Method steps, 56, 57
    when to present, 74–75
    writing as group, 69*f*
Seating arrangements for groups, 61
Self-acceptance, *see* Ego integrity versus
    despair
Self-consciousness, 35
Self-efficacy, 33–34
Self-esteem
    art activities and, 158
    gerotranscendence and, 149
    intrinsic motivation and, 28, 33, 115,
        119
Self-expression, 67
Self-growth, 122–123
Self/identity, 132–133, 147
Sensory cortex, 91, 91*f*
    see also Brain stimulation and TTAP
        Method steps
Sensory stimulation
    cognitive reserve and, 95
    importance of, 88–89
    intergenerational programming in,
        83–84
    learning style/brain regions and, 108*t,*
        118*f*

overview of, 56, 79–80
see also TTAP Method steps
Sequence patterns, 49, 50*f*
Session attendance and duration,
    160–161, 160*f*
Severe/late-stage Alzheimer's disease
    description of, 9, 10*f*, 15, 23
    life review and, 131
    therapeutic recreation and, 127
    TTAP Method steps and, *see*
        Severe/late-stage Alzheimer's
        disease and TTAP Method steps
Severe/late-stage Alzheimer's disease and
    TTAP Method steps
    conversation, 71
    drama/theater, 80
    food experiences and, 73
    movement/dance, 68
    music/meditation, 57
    phototherapy, 78
    reaching out/involvement and, 76
    sculpture, 64–65
    sensory stimulation, 79–80
    theme events, 75–76
Social relationships
    artistic imagery process and, 113
    benefits of, 29, 30*f*, 39, 46
    Continuum of Psychological Domains
        and, 130
    Levine Madori Taxonomy and, 153,
        154*f*
    person-centered care and, 161
    TTAP Method benefits to, 119, 158
Spatial learners, 106*t*
Spatial relations, 12
Spirituality, 130, 154*f*
Staff and TTAP Method benefits, 170
Stimulation, *see* Brain stimulation;
    Cognitive stimulation; Memory
    stimulation; Sensory stimulation
Storytelling, 37–38, 70
Strategic system, 107, 107*b*, 109
Strengths of adults with Alzheimer's
    disease, 29–31, 30*f*, 109–110, 110*f*, 136
Stress and cognition, 100
Styles of learning, 105–108, 106*t*, 108*t*,
    115, 116*t*–117*t*
Synapses, 7
Synthesis level, 104–105

Tangles, neurofibrillary, 96–97, 98–99
Taxonomies, 103–105, 149–155, 150*f*,
    151*f*, 153*f*, 154*f*

TCI, *see* Theme-centered interaction
    theory
Temporal lobe, 91, 91*f*, 169*f*
see also Brain stimulation and TTAP
    Method steps
Theater, *see* Drama or theater
Theme(s)
    benefits of, 27–28, 145–146
    cognitive/brain stimulation and,
        107–110, 108*t*, 110*f*
    communication and, 138
    Continuum of Psychological Domains
        and, 127–131, 128*t*
    emergence of, 61
    events, *see* Theme events
    graphic organizing tools for, 48–49,
        50*f*, 51
    life review and, 133–134, 134*f*
    object relations theory and, 142*f*
    theme-centered interaction and, 144*f*,
        145, 146
    see also specific names of themes
Theme-centered interaction theory (TCI),
    143–146, 144*f*
Theme events
    brain stimulation and, 76, 107–110,
        108*t*, 110*f*, 118*f*
    intergenerational programming in,
        83
    overview of, 55, 73–76, 74*f*
    see also TTAP Method steps
Theories underlying TTAP Method
    Continuum of Psychological
        Domains, 127–131, 128*t*
    developmental theories, 122–126,
        127
    gerotranscendence, 146–149
    humanistic psychology, 135–138
    life review and, 131–135, 134*f*
    life-span theory, 124–126
    neurodevelopmental theory/
        treatment, 138–140, 140*f*
    object relations theory, 141, 142*b*,
        142*f*, 143
    person-centered care and, 121
    theme-centered interaction theory
        (TCI), 143–146, 144*f*
    therapeutic recreation and, 126–127
Therapeutic recreation, 126–127
Therapeutic recreation specialists, 43–44
Therapeutic storytelling, 37–38, 70
Therapeutic Thematic Arts Programming
    Method, *see* TTAP Method

Time
    communication about, 16*f*, 17, 18*f*
    confusion of, 12, 14
    creative process and, 112
    flow and, 35
Tracking, *see* Documentation of research
    on TTAP Method
Transcendence, 153–155, 154*f*
TTAP Method
    benefits of, *see* TTAP Method benefits
    CCDERS Approach and, 29–31, 30*f*,
        32*f*, 84–85
    communication and, 46–48
    concept application, 31, 33–38
    dual focus of, 113
    foundations of, *see* Brain stimulation;
        Learning and intelligence; Theories
        underlying TTAP Method
    as multimodal care approach, 38–39
    objectives of, 25, 26, 32*f*, 56
    steps of, *see* TTAP Method steps
    strengths/abilities and, 13
    themes in, 27–28
TTAP Method benefits
    brain plasticity, 138–139, 140, 140*f*
    brain stimulation, 87, 109–110, 110*f*,
        111
    CCDERS Approach, 29–31, 30*f*, 32*f*,
        84–85
    client feedback on, 115, 119, 158, 163
    creative process and, 111–112
    documentation of, *see* Documentation
        of research on TTAP Method
    gerotranscendence, 148–149
    individualized thematic
        programming, 27, 145–146
    life review, 133–134, 134*f*
    to memory, 166, 167*f*, 168
    moderate Alzheimer's and, 115, 119
    monetary impact on facility, 170
    to mood, 164*f*, 165
    object relations, 143
    overview of, 25–26, 33, 40, 41,
        84–85, 155, 170–171
    person-centered care, 137–138
    transcendence, 154–155, 154*f*
    see also Alzheimer's disease delay/
        prevention; *specific benefits*
TTAP Method steps
    Alzheimer's stages and, *see specific
        Alzheimer's stages*
    benefits of, 31
    Bloom's Taxonomy in, 152

    brain stimulation and, *see* Brain
        stimulation and TTAP Method steps
    client feedback/evaluation, 56, 80–82
    communication as first, 46–48
    conversation, 54, 56–57
    drama/theater, 56, 80
    drawing/painting, 55, 59–62, 59*f*, 62*f*
    food experiences, 55, 71–73, 72*f*
    gerotranscendence and, 148–149
    intergenerational programming in,
        82–84
    learning style/brain region and,
        107–108, 108*t*, 115, 116*t*–117*t*
    movement/dance, 55, 65–68, 65*f*
    multimodal approach of, 40
    music/meditation, 55, 57, 58*b*
    object relations theory and, 141,
        142*b*, 142*f*, 143
    overview of, 28–29, 54–56
    phototherapy, 55, 76–78, 77*f*
    sculpture, 55, 63–65, 63*f*, 64*f*
    sensory stimulation, 56, 79–80
    theme-centered interaction theory
        (TCI) and, 146
    theme events, 55, 73–76, 74*f*
    theories underlying, 134–135
    writing in groups, 37–38, 55, 68–71,
        69*f*, 70*f*
    see also specific steps
TTAP Method with Alzheimer's disease
    benefits of, 158, 163
    common problems addressed, 44–46
    descriptive patterning, 48–49, 50*f*, 51
    gerotranscendence and, 149
    graphic organizing tools, 51–53
    Levine Madori Taxonomy and,
        153–155, 153*f*, 154*f*
    as multimodal care approach, 38–39
    person-centered care, 137–138
    procedural memory stimulation,
        53–54
    steps in, 54–56
    therapists needed for, 43–44
    see also Alzheimer's disease delay/
        prevention; *specific Alzheimer's stages*

Understanding level, 150*f*, 151, 151*f*, 152,
    153*f*

Verbal expression, 161
    see also Communication; Language
Very mild cognitive decline stage, 21
Very severe cognitive decline stage, 24

Visual images, 12
    see also Guided imagery and music

Well-being, 25, 80–81
Wellness
    activity participation and, 125
    ego integrity and, 123
    flow and, 111–112
    therapeutic recreation and, 126
Wernicke's area, 91*f*, 93, 169*f*
    see also Brain stimulation and TTAP
        Method steps
Windows into past interests, 121
Windows of lucidity, 45–46

Withdrawal
    Alzheimer's disease and, 12–13, 15, 22
    communication breakdown and, 17*f*
    excess disability and, 101
    prevention of progression and, 16
Words as therapy, 37–38
Writing as group
    brain stimulation and, 71, 108*t*, 117*t*,
        169*f*
    graphic organizing tools and, 51, 52
    intergenerational programming in,
        82–83
    overview of, 37–38, 55, 68–71, 69*f*, 70*f*
    see also TTAP Method steps